Dietger Mathias

Diet and exercise
Current medical knowledge on how to keep healthy

Fit from
1 to 100

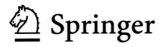 Springer

Dietger Mathias, M.D., D.Sc.
Augasse 7A
69207 Sandhausen

ISBN 978-3-662-49194-2

The German National Library documents this publication in the German National Bibliography; detailed bibliographic data are accessible in the Internet via http://dnb.d-nb.de.

Springer
© Springer-Verlag Berlin Heidelberg 2016

Cover illustration: © D. Mathias (private)
Translated by: Deborah Ann Landry, Landry & Associates International, Göttingen, Germany

Printed on acid-free and chlorine-free bleached paper.

Springer-Verlag GmbH Berlin Heidelberg, Part of Springer Science+Business Media (www.springer.com)
(www.springer.com)

Diet and exercise
Current medical knowledge on how to keep healthy

Fit from 1 to 100

For Lilly and Lucy

Table of Content

II Exercise

III Appendix

Lateral growth as a result of maldevelopment in early childhood – A preface

The factors decisive in leading a healthy lifestyle include eating a varied diet, taking plenty of exercise, not smoking and practicing judicious restraint when it comes to drinking alcoholic beverages. It is important to start the education and information process about these facts at an early age. Indeed, children retain these teachings when they turn into adults. Unfortunately, the necessary learning processes fall by the wayside all too often, thereby making childhood maldevelopment an inevitable outcome.

Nearly 22 million children and adolescents living in the European Union are overweight. In one of the more affluent and industrialized countries like Germany alone, this can be said about nearly 2 million of the 3 to 17-year-olds. Around 800,000 of them have already become obese. Every year, over 200 of these fat adolescents in Germany develop adult-onset diabetes. Large international studies have consistently confirmed that adolescents who are too heavy already tend to contract coronary heart disease and cancer in addition to diabetes during middle age at a much greater frequency than their age-matched normal-weight counterparts (▶ Chapter 37). In the USA, the proportion of children suffering from chronic conditions due to morbid obesity nearly doubled over a 12-year period (van Cleave et al. 2010). Close to 17 % of the children and adolescents aged 2 and 19 years living there are obese (Ogden et al. 2012).

The German adolescents who are too fat spend on average 23 hours a day just lying down, sitting or standing. Four out of five 15-year-olds are no longer capable of balancing themselves while moving two or more steps backwards. Nine out of ten cannot stand on one leg for longer than a minute. However, early childhood is when and where the desire and capability to be physically activity starts and actually persists for a long time thereafter. Hence, there are also hardly any limitations in terms of movement competence, even in children up to the age of 6. The problems start around the age of 10 years and become clearly evident in 15-year-olds. In many countries, the children nowadays are around 15 % less fit than their parents were 30 years ago (Tomkinson 2013). That is one reason why exercise training assumes an increasingly important role. At best, it should be initiated in preschoolers. For older children and adolescents, at least one hour of strenuous exercise per day is recommended. Besides its intensity, kinetic variety in exercise plays a pivotal role.

Athletic school children often achieve better overall grades than their "couch potato" counterparts in their age group: That means they get off to a more successful start in their professional lives (Kantomaa et al. 2013, Booth et al. 2014). Because the majority of children then continue to practice sports as adults, they are thereby also sustainably enhancing their quality of life and will benefit over the long term from the many positive health effects emanating from their physical activity. The same similarly applies to stress situations they encounter later in life. In such situations, people usually subconsciously fall back into their old habits. That is when it is beneficial to fall back on good accustomed habits like practicing sports or eating a sensible diet (Neal et al. 2013).

1 Introduction

According to the findings of the Global Burden of Disease Study, 2.1 billion people worldwide are too fat. Since 1980, the magnitude of this problem has grown by 28 % in adults and by as much as 47 % in children (Ng et al. 2014). In Germany, a study on adults' health showed that 53 % of women and 67 % of men are overweight, with 24 % of women and 23 % of men suffering from obesity (Mensink et al. 2013).

Because physical activity and a sensible diet positively impact a person's well-being and health, incentivizing personal initiative and self-responsibility is essential for promoting sensible lifestyles. Obviously, a diet consisting of plenty of fruit and vegetables, but restraint when it comes to eating meat, and a lifestyle that includes physical activity at least 2.5 hours a week, while avoiding obesity and refraining from the use of tobacco will all lower the risk for serious diseases like diabetes, cancer, myocardial infarction and stroke by more than half (Ford et al. 2009, Rasmussen et al. 2013). Another large-scale study on a cohort of 20,900 men and women showed that positive assessment of the lifestyle factors exercise, body weight, sufficient consumption of breakfast cereals, fruits and vegetables, non-smoking and only moderate alcohol intake lowered the risk of heart failure (Djousse et al. 2009). And the key result from investigations on 83,882 women presented by the Nurses' Health Study (▶ Chapter 3) was a reduction in the prevalence of hypertension by 80 % in women who were not overweight, engaged in 30 minutes of physical activity a week and ate a healthy diet (Forman et al. 2009).

That means that it is becoming increasingly helpful for people to be provided with the most com-prehensive knowledge on this subject as possible. Namely, if precise knowledge of the facts shapes our thoughts, then the danger that a poorly balanced diet and lack of exercise will shape the body is lower. The more comprehensive their knowledge of the facts is, the easier people can be compelled to modify their lifestyles and the greater becomes the likelihood that their modified lifestyles will be associated with a permanently successful outcome. It is especially important to begin intensively fostering an aware-ness for a health-promoting lifestyle in children at a young age. This is when they are impressionable and not biased or predisposed. They readily assimilate the principles of good behavior, while no bad habits have been reinforced yet. In addition to the parents, this is also the mission of kindergartens and schools. The prevailing advertising ban imposed by the food industry aimed to protect children under 12 years of age must be complied with unconditionally and with no room for impunity.

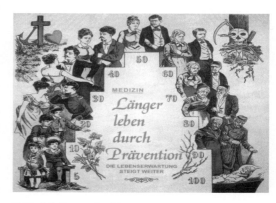

◼ **Fig. 1.1** Source: dpa/akg

I Diet

2 "Who doesn't know anything, has to believe everything."

Marie von Ebner-Eschenbach (1830 – 1916), often attributed to Albert Einstein (1879–1955)

Knowledge about the fundamentals of nutrition and diet always confers great benefit. In order to be able to reap these benefits over the long term, habits associated with deep emotions must be added into the equation. It is a given that eating is more than just the intake of food: Eating involves retrospection, ritual, entertainment, often reward – and sometimes it is even an ordeal. However, if we succeed in steering the acquired knowledge along the path of reason, this will most likely also have the desired sustainable effects on health as well.

The physical and psychological harms caused by overweight and obesity are enormous. Approximately one-third of all cancer cases alone can be attributed to the wrong diet. That means that healthy people are not only happier. Indeed, the sounder the knowledge each individual has about health issues, the greater is the added value for our economy. First of all, well-found knowledge can protect against the often high-priced, but useless pseudo-medicinal products offered. Secondly, the constant progress made in all fields of medicine also makes the healthcare system more and more expensive. In 2012, an aggregate of € 300.4 billion was spent on healthcare, € 185 billion (= 61.4 %) of this was spent within the German statutory health insurance scheme. By comparison, the total budget of the Federal Republic of Germany runs at € 306 billion. Treatments for diet-related diseases incur annual costs of approximately € 100 billion. And because the growth in medical knowledge keeps increasing at such a fast pace, the state of the art will no longer be exclusively affordable through fixed health insurance premiums. Over the long or the short: **prevention** is always a sensible financial investment in the future for everyone.

Moreover, the age structure in our society is constantly changing. Ever more people are reaching very old age. According to data from the German Federal Office of Statistics, one in three inhabitants of the Federal Republic of Germany will be over the age of 60 by the year 2030. According to the World Health Organization (WHO), the proportion of individuals in this age group is growing the fastest in almost every country. Viewed from the angle of healthy aging, the financial viability of our healthcare systems assumes an every greater role. Better programs for promoting healthy lifestyle are therefore very important. A general acceptance of them exists. In our times of growing and more prevalent affluence, attitudes towards health take on new dimensions. Surveys have repeatedly confirmed that health is rated as the most valuable commodity.

3   Pivotal long-term studies

Even the greatest nonsense purported is frequently justified by the fact that there was a study on it. In the field of **nutrition** alone, approximately 9000 articles are published in the medical literature worldwide every year – that is close to one "study" per hour. Reference to such nutritional studies therefore does not necessarily pack that much weight, especially when obviously backed by an interest group from industry. In contrast, the results from recognized research groups working at renowned universities or institutes published in specialized journals with high impact factors are much more compelling (Appendix). Here, the large-scale, international interventional and monitoring trials enrolling tens of thousands of volunteers and lasting many years should be given particular emphasis (◘ Tab. 3.1). Even their findings cannot automatically be assigned the conclusiveness given to laws of Nature, but they do constantly and reliably improve our knowledge about the many details of the physiological interconnections between diet, exercise and health. These form the basis of the content of the following chapters.

Among others, one of the most scientifically sound pieces of research is the **Framingham Heart Study**. On April 12, 1945, President Franklin D. Roosevelt died unexpectedly of a stroke. This event triggered the worldwide-longest, still ongoing study of cardiovascular disease. The town of Framingham with its 28,000 inhabitants in the area of Boston Massachusetts was chosen as the study site. The town's inhabitants were regarded as representing the perfect cross-section of the American population. This study is now investigating the third generation, usually comprising around 5000 test subjects.

◘ **Tab. 3.1** Examples of major prospective long-term studies

Study	Ongoing since	Number of subjects
Black Women's Health Study	1995	59,000
California Teachers Study	1995	133,400
Cancer Prevention Study	1960 (to 1972)	1 million
Cancer Prevention Study II	1982	1.2 millions
Cancer Prevention Study III	2010	500,000
EPIC Study	1992	519,000
Framingham Heart Study	1948	5000
Health Professionals Follow-up Study	1986	51,500
Interheart Study	1997	30,000
NIH-AARP Diet and Health Study	1995	567,000
Nurses' Health Study I	1976	122,000
Nurses' Health Study II	1989	116,500
Procam Study	1978	50,000
Whitehall II Study	1985	10,300
Women's Health Initiative	1991	161,800

4 The human body – a giant chemical factory

Today's lifestyle-related illnesses frequently originate from the change that has occurred in the everyday lives of teenagers. The loss of playing on the streets because of traffic-clogged street, the disappearance of other space for free movement and the magnetic draw of electronic media are major causes of this phenomenon. Nutrient deficiencies relating to a misinterpretation of the optimized combination of foods and the high proclivity for eating fast food have continued to drive down the deterioration of people's health further.

That said, our body can be regarded as one giant complex and complicated chemical factory, consisting of approximately 10^{28} atoms. The mean atomic weight of these basic building blocks for our body is assumed to be 4.5 g (per approx. 6×10^{23} atoms). The genome works as the supreme regulator of all functions. Its 3 billion DNA base pairs which reside in the 23 chromosomes make it very large. Each chromosome contains genes which carry the instructions for making proteins – the function bearers of the body's cells. The currently known human genome catalog contains some 21,000 protein-encoding genes (Neumann et al. 2010). Terminologically analogous to the genome, the set of proteins our body produces from them in its tissue is called the proteome. To date, a good 90 % of our proteome has been identified (Kim et al. 2014, Wilhelm et al. 2014).

These proteins include, e.g. numerable structural proteins with long half-lives. However, many isoforms exist, like enzyme proteins, messenger substances of the immune system or the plasma cells, which produce up to 10,000 antibodies per second and are reproduced every day. And these are just several notable examples of the thousands of other chemical reactions for which the proper substitute substances have to be constantly replenished through our food.

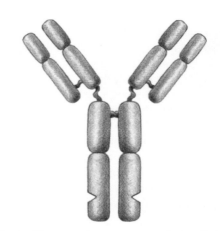

◘ **Fig. 4.1** Diagrammatic representation of an antibody molecule

5   Our food – an energy transfer medium

The desirable nutritional percentages for energy transfer carried by the macronutrients are
- carbohydrates: approx. 55–60 %,
- fats: approx. 30 %,
- 1/3 saturated fatty acids,
- 1/3 monounsaturated fatty acids, e.g. oleic acid,
- 1/3 polyunsaturated fatty acids
  (► Chapter 15),
- Proteins: approximately 10 % (approx. 0.8–1 g/kg body weight). Children and adolescents require roughly 15 % protein a day.

Essential amino acids the body cannot synthesize are: Isoleucine, leucine, lysine, methionine, phenylalanine, threonine, tryptophan and valine.

The ratio of amino acids in ingested proteins should as closely as possible equal the composition of the proteins in the body. In other words, the biological value placed on proteins should be high. This applies to most animal protein, especially to milk, eggs, fish and meat. By contrast, some vegetable proteins do contain individual amino acids, albeit only in relatively low amounts.

The biological value of several proteins (in percent):
- Milk 100
- Whole egg 93
- Potato 92
- Beef 85
- Fish 83
- Rice 75
- Rye flour 74
- Peas 52
- Corn 22

The primary objective of food intake is supplying energy to the cells and tissues, whereby fats, carbohydrates and proteins can replace one another to a large extent. The energy stored in the form of carbohydrates is limited to 400–450 g, approximately 350 g in muscles and 80 g in the liver. As energy suppliers, proteins are less relevant under normal conditions. It is not until food becomes scarce that proteins start to play a role. This is because several amino acids are convertible into glucose. All excess energy derived from the food eaten is stored in the body's adipose tissue. In the case of fat, only 3 % of the calories eaten are necessary for this storage process. By contrast, carbohydrates must first be converted to fat – a process that burns up as much as almost 25 % of the calories consumed.

According to the fundamental principles of physics, all 3 caloric sources – when consumed in excess – are responsible for lateral growth. But because fat contains more than twice as high a proportion of energy as carbohydrates or proteins do, limiting the body's fat intake is a particularly effective way to maintain or achieve one's desired weight.

6 Energy production

In the cells, energy production starts with a series of reactions called the **citric acid cycle** which requires the building block **pyruvate** from the breakdown of carbohydrates to work. If pyruvate becomes scarce because, e.g. the limited carbohydrate stores have been emptied by strong physical exertion, then the metabolism of fats (and proteins) only takes place to a very limited extent (▸ Chapter 7).

As much as 10 % of the adenosine triphosphate molecules (ATP) necessary for the functional processes of the cells to work are generated in the citric acid cycle. The other 90 % are then produced by oxidative phosphorylation in the respiratory chain, closely linked to the citric acid cycle. The efficiency with which the chemical energy of nutrients can be converted into functional ATP in these processes is only approximately 43 %. The large proportion of this energy flows into heat generation (▸ Chapter 9 and ▸ Chapter 71).

> Carbohydrates ignite the flame that burns fats.

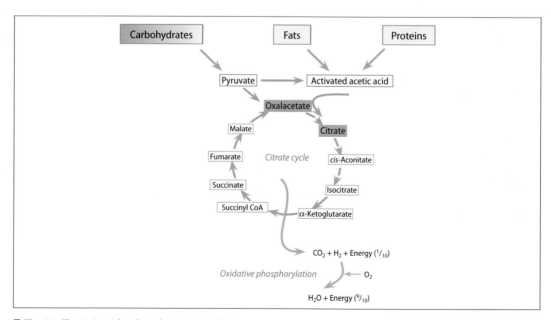

◘ **Fig. 6.1** The citric acid cycle and respiratory chain

7   Energy production when food is scarce

Although glucose is being consumed constantly by the body, the blood glucose levels remain constant during limited fasting, e. g. at night, thanks to the action of glucagon. Three-quarters of the glucose converted by the liver under these conditions comes from glycogen and the rest is synthesized by gluconeogenesis. If the body goes from a state of temporary abstinence from food into a fasting state, the adaptation processes of the body's metabolism are potentiated. This is imperative given that the glycogen reserves in the liver only last for barely 24 hours when the body is at rest. Afterwards, the blood glucose levels start to gradually drop to within approximately 2/3 of the normal range, but may not fall below 40 mg/100 ml because otherwise the brain would stop functioning. The red blood corpuscles and the adrenal medulla, for example, are strictly dependent on glucose for "fuel".

Fatty acids cannot be converted into glucose. Amino acids are available as alternatives for the synthesis of glucose. But for that, the body must sacrifice its protein. This response can only represent a stopgap solution for the body given that as much as 2 g of protein are necessary for the synthesis of 1 g of glucose and the fact that a prolonged loss of protein would cause considerable organic damage to the body. Because of the toll that fasting takes on energy utilization, all adaptation mechanisms tend to steer away from carbohydrates and more towards the fats and ketone bodies. The latter include acetone, acetoacetic acid and 3-hydroxybutyric acid. After approximately 3 days of starvation, these are produced in the liver from the breakdown of fat. In other words, they can be understood as the easy-to-transport energy equivalents of fatty acids. As needed, and after a short adaptation phase, the brain can even absorb them and use them as a main source of energy.

Acetoacetic acid and hydroxybutyric acid help to elevate the concentration of hydrogen ions in the blood. This, in turn, also stimulates the kidneys to produce glucose, primarily from the amino acid glutamine.

This rate is considerably below that of 130 g/day, the rate of nocturnal fasting. But due to the capability of the brain to switch from burning glucose to burning ketone bodies, endogenous protein remains mostly spared here.

> Over a longer fasting period, the liver and kidneys ultimately produce a total of 80 g glucose a day, with each organ doing approximately half of this work.

8 Energy expenditure I – basal metabolic rate

Even when completely at rest, the body requires a minimum amount of energy to perform the minimal amount of bodily activity, regulate body temperature and sustain the various cell functions. Under normal daily exertion, this basal metabolic rate accounts for approximately two thirds of the body's total energy expenditure. Nearly 80 % of this is distributed among
- brain (18 %),
- heart (9 %),
- skeletal muscle (26 %) and
- liver (26 %).

The basal metabolic rate is an inconstant variable, it correlates closely with the lean body mass (= total weight minus weight of adipose tissues). At a normal body mass index (▶ Chapter 38), this so-called lean mass makes up around 75 % of the body weight in women and 80 % in men. When athletic persons gain weight, the basal metabolic rate increases by approx. 3 kilocalories (kcal) per kilogram (kg) of lean mass per day. But if the weight increase only involves enlarging the fatty padding, the basal metabolic rate will hardly change. That is another reason why only minor weight losses can be achieved over the medium term by diet alone in persons who are physically inactive.

With increasing age, the metabolic processes slow down and muscle strength becomes weaker – one explanation for why the elderly have a lower basal metabolic rate than young people (▶ Chapter 77). The approximately 10 % larger muscle mass of men compared to women means that males of the species have a higher basal metabolic rate of around 5 %. During sleep, the basal metabolic rate drops by 7–10 %, during longer periods of fasting by 20–40 %. Stress, sweating, fever and living in regions with low temperatures all elevate this rate while depression and acclimation to tropical temperatures, for example, lower it.

The variables impacting the basal metabolic rate are primarily controlled by the **thyroid hormones**. They crank up oxygen consumption and cause an increase in **thermogenesis** (▶ Chapter 9). By contrast, in persons dieting, thyroid hormones active in regulatory processes are secreted in reduced concentrations. The basal metabolic rate is throttled by the associated restriction in heat production. In earlier times of shortage, this physiologically sensible adaptation mechanism enabled the individual's survival time to be prolonged, whereas nowadays it encumbers weight loss in candidates seeking to adhere to a disciplined diet.

> The average basal metabolic rate of a 25-year-old woman runs at around 1.0 kcal (4 kJ) per kg body weight and hour; in a 25-year-old man it is approximately 1.1 kcal (4.4 kJ).

9   Energy expenditure II – heat production

In principal, heat is generated as a by-product of the energy produced to maintain the body's basal and active metabolic rates (▶ Chapter 8 and ▶ Chapter 10). By steering metabolism, the iodine-containing thyroid hormones work as the main regulators of heat production. This process mainly takes place in the muscles, although heat generation is also possible in the fatty tissue. Here, we must differentiate between white tissue and brown tissue: Thermogenesis primarily takes place in brown adipose tissue (BAT). To date, this has only been unequivocally detectable at higher concentrations in neonates in their first days of life. The additional heat produced by this fat protects babies against cold. However, because this BAT rapidly undergoes involution with increasing age, it stops playing any major functional role for a long time. BAT is endowed with a rich blood and nerve supply, while refined techniques have meanwhile been developed that can detect minor – sometimes even larger – amounts of this tissue along the great arteries in adults (Lee et al. 2013).

In the mitochondria of this specialized tissue is where uncoupling protein-1 (UCP1, **thermogenin**) resides. Other uncoupling proteins (UCPs) can be found in skeletal muscle and white adipose tissue.

Thermogenin especially, but also the other UCPs, cut off the flow of hydrogen ions at the inner mitochondrial membrane. This process is initiated by noradrenaline. Here, it reacts with a β-receptor coupled to a G protein and results in defective adenosine triphosphate (ATP) synthesis (▶ Chapter 6).

Nevertheless, ATP is the actual driver of energy metabolism in the body. To a certain degree, it is the "electric current" essentially enabling all vital processes in cells to run at all. Therefore, ATP must always be rapidly produced in adequate amounts from carbohydrates and fats. However, if ATP synthesis is inhibited, more of the consumed dietary energy is directed to this important process, with the result that heat release increases and a possible energy surplus is less likely to be stored in the form of fat. Some individuals benefit from the energy-consuming properties of UCPs to a greater extent because they produce more of such proteins. The disturbance of biological processes caused thereby allows those affected to apparently eat as much as they want and still remain slim. This unique characteristic of a metabolism that constantly overproduces heat is also referred to as **"non-exercise activity thermogenesis"**.

10 Energy expenditure III – active metabolic rate

For each additional task that a person performs above and beyond the body's basal metabolic rate – be it muscular or concentrated brain activity – the active metabolic rate factors into the equation. Lighter activities consume 0.5–1 kcal per hour per kg of body weight, moderate activities 1–2 kcal, strenuous activities 2–12 kcal and considerably strenuous activities consume more than 12 kcal per hour per kg of body weight. In everyday life, these values are reflected in the recommendations, for example like those issued by the German Nutrition Society, which set daily caloric intake targets based on muscular activity. In persons aged between 25 and 50 years with normal body mass index (BMI) and average physical activity, for example, the general range is set at 2300 kcal per day for women and 2900 kcal for men (❏ Tab. 10.1). For reference, the type of work performed by homemakers, restaurant servers or handymen is defined as moderate physical activity.

Caloric expenditure increases in people who additionally take regular exercise in their leisure time. This increase in caloric consumption often assumes significant proportions, as the data from some professional athletes show. For such athletes, however, time can be a limiting factor when it comes to eating the "mountains" of food they need to meet their energy demands, especially since vigorous physical activity generally has an appetite-reducing effect that lasts for 1–2 hours afterwards. This phenomenon can be observed, for instance, in cyclists who participate in long-distance road races. Today's high-energy drinks help athletes cope with this specific problem.

❏ **Tab. 10.1** Reference values for daily energy input in persons with a normal BMI and an average level of physical activity

Age (years)	Basal metabolic rate plus active metabolic rate			
	Male		Female	
	kcal	kJ	kcal	kJ
15–18	3100	12,400	2,500	10,000
19–24	3,000	12,000	2,400	9,600
25–50	2,900	11,600	2,300	9,200
51–65	2,500	10,000	2,000	8,000
≥65	2,300	9,200	1,800	7,200

BMI Body Mass Index, *kcal* Kilocalorie, *kJ* Kilojoule

11 Physical activity level

For reasons of uniformity, it has become common international practice to represent the average daily energy requirement for physical activity as a proportion of the basal metabolic rate. Accordingly, this measure of metabolic energy requirements is called the **"physical activity level" (PAL)**.

> PAL = total energy expenditure/
> basal metabolic rate (TEE/BMR)

The advantage of this approach is that certain factors influencing energy requirements such as age, gender and body weight are already factored into the equation, thus enabling us to compare the energy expenditure for defined physical activities in different types of people. The daily energy expend-

iture is estimated by multiplying the duration of the individual activities by the value for the respective basal metabolic rate (Yamada et al. 2013, Westerterp 2013).

As an example, a 24-hour period comprising 8 hours of work with a high energy requirement of 2.4 PAL, 8 hours of work with an average energy expenditure of 1.6 PAL and 8 hours of sleep with 0.95 PAL, adds up to a PAL of

$$(2.4 \times 8 + 1.6 \times 8 + 0.95 \times 8) : 24 = \mathbf{1.65}$$

In persons engaging in athletic activities totaling 3–5 hours per week, 0.3 PAL units per day can be added to the respectively calculated values. ◻ Tab. 11.1 lists some of the PAL values describing common activities as formulated by the German Nutrition Society.

◻ **Tab. 11.1** Energy expenditure for various activities measured by basal metabolic rate

Type of physical activity	PAL	Examples
Heavy occupational work	2.0–2.4	Construction workers, farmers, high performance athletes
Predominantly standing or walking work	1.8–1.9	Homemakers, salespersons, restaurant servers, mechanics, traders
Sedentary activity/seated work with some requirement for occasional walking or standing work	1.6–1.7	Drivers, laboratory assistants, students
seated work with little or no strenuous leisure activity	1.4–1.5	Office employees, precision mechanics
Exclusively sedentary or bedridden lifestyle	1.2	Old, infirm individuals
Sleep	0.95	

PAL Physical Activity Level

12 Control of energy metabolism in the brain

The brain regulates energy expenditure by means of hunger and satiety. The hypothalamus, a part of the diencephalon, plays a key role in this highly complex process (Vaag 2009, Nguyen et al. 2011). The hormones **neuropeptide Y (NPY)** and **Agouti-related protein (AGRP)** stimulate appetite and reduce energy consumption in the basal metabolic rate. Antagonists of NPY and AGRP are the **α-melanocyte-stimulating hormone (α-MSH)** as well as the **cocaine and amphetamine-regulated transcript (CART)**. Both curb appetite and increase energy consumption. NPY/AGRP thus act like a gas pedal on our appetite and α-MSH/CART like a brake.

These systems initially mutually inhibit each other, while normal glucose levels act to regulate these processes. Declining glucose concentrations coupled with insufficient dietary intake, however, cancel out the inhibitory effect of the αMSH/CART cell group. The now predominantly NPY/AGRP system stimulates the production of **orexins A** and **B,** which trigger hunger in the lateral hypothalamus. In addition, these activate the "wake" function of the brain. After all, one has to be awake to want to consume or, as was imperative in former times, go out and forage for food. After satiety has been reached, the glucose molecules now present at higher concentrations displace the orexins of their receptors. The appetite diminishes, the person gets tired and can fall asleep better.

The insidious trap in this context, however, is today's exaggerated consumption of pure sugar, e. g. reflected in the frequent imbibing of soft drinks, which many start early in childhood (► Chapter 45). Indeed, only half of normal granulated sugar con-

sists of glucose. The other half is fructose. Although fructose delivers the same number of calories as glucose, it does not act like a brake to intervene in the signaling controls of energy metabolism like glucose does (► Chapter 14). That is why these sugar-sweetened beverages can very rapidly cause fat to accumulate in the body (Caprio 2012, de Ruyter et al. 2012, Te Morenga et al. 2013, Page et al. 2013).

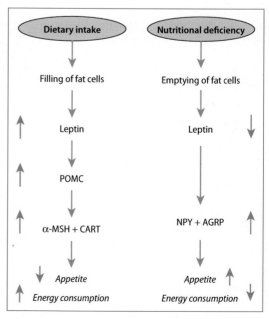

◘ **Fig. 12.1** Regulation of appetite and energy expenditure. *POMC* Proopiomelanocortin, *red arrow* reduction, *blue arrow* increase

13 Control of energy metabolism by endogenous hormones

There are important endogenous hormones that also interact closely with and regulate the hypothalamic control system. One of them is **leptin**. Discovered in 1994, it plays a crucial role in this signaling cascade. Leptin is produced in the lipocytes in direct relation to the fat being stored there. At higher concentrations, this 167 amino-acid adipocytokine activates the appetite-suppressing α-MSH/CART peptides and, at lower concentrations, stimulates the appetite-stimulating hormones NPY and AGRP. Hence, a rise or increase in leptin levels in the body is able to switch the hypothalamic hunger centers on and off. Unlike glucose, leptin is chiefly responsible for achieving a long-term energy balance over weeks.

Ghrelin is another important endogenous hormone that helps regulate how nutritional intake is absorbed by the body. It is primarily produced in the stomach and pancreas and stimulates the sensation of hunger. This stimulation disappears when the stomach is full.

Glucagon-like peptide-1, synthesized in the small intestine, amplifies the "appetite-braking" response to a full stomach because it slows the emptying of gastric contents into the intestine. Post-prandial stomach wall stretching is an additional signal for cholecystokinin. This polypeptide hormone is secreted in the intestine and inhibits the appetite-triggering hormones NPY and AGRP, thereby suppressing the urge to eat (▶ Chapter 44). Peptide YY3-36 works in the same way. Depending on caloric intake, Peptide YY3-36 is secreted in the large intestine after meals.

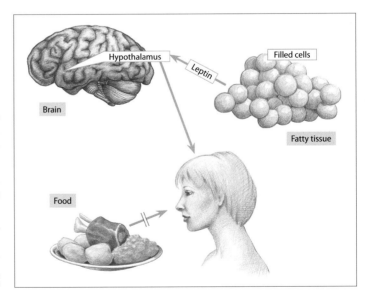

▣ **Fig. 13.1** Leptin suppresses the appetite

14 Control of energy metabolism – the reward system

Most people define nutrition in rather archaic terms, using the verbs to eat, drink and enjoy. Catch phrases like dining culture, culinary arts, delicacies, sumptuous spreads and feasting all give testimony to the high value our society places on people giving into their urge to eat. In fact, eating well contributes to life's enjoyment and when partaken of in moderation, can improve the state of our health merely by uplifting our psyche.

That said, our eating behavior is also strongly influenced by the people close to us. According to a long-term evaluation as part of the Framingham Heart Study, which repeatedly assessed a densely interconnected social network of 12,067 people from 1971 to 2003, there was a 57 % probability that a person would become overweight if their boyfriend or girlfriend had become overweight during the same period. The same probability was 40 % for siblings and 37 % for married couples. These effects did not transfer to other people in their immediate neighborhood. Genome analyses have also shown that very good friends exhibit hemophilic genotypes (Christakis et Fowler 2007, 2014).

Responsibility for the psychological effects of dietary intake has now been primarily attributed to the endogenous cannabinoids, discovered to modulate the feedback loops involved in hypothalamic appetite regulation via the specific endocannabinoid receptor CB1. The **endocannabinoids** are part of a reward system in the brain, which explains

their secretion after a well-tasting meal is consumed or food intake occurs after a period of fasting. Under normal conditions, this process is designed to maintain an energy balance. However, frequent excessive food intake leads to long-term overregulation of the endocannabinoid system, the consequence being an incessant craving for food and the consumption of increasingly large quantities thereof. This phenomenon is accompanied by a simultaneous further increase in endogenous cannabinoid levels (► Chapter 35). The administration of the anti-obesity drug rimonabant (tradename Acomplia) has been shown to break this vicious circle by medically blocking the CB1 receptor. However, the drug was taken off the European market in autumn of 2008 because of its strong psychological side effects.

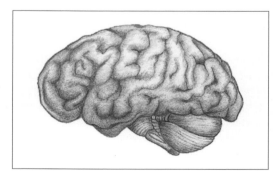

◘ Fig. 14.1

15 Unsaturated fatty acids

Fatty acids are long-chain hydrocarbons. They are called unsaturated fatty acids when they lack the maximum possible number of hydrogen atoms attached to every carbon atom. For example, if stearic acid, which has 18 carbon atoms and frequently occurs in animal and plant fats, is missing 2 hydrogen atoms, then a double bond is present and the resulting acid is oleic acid. Its polyunsaturated derivatives **linoleic acid (omega-6)** and **linolenic acid (omega-3)** have 2 and 3 double bonds, respectively. Omega-3 and omega-6 fatty acids are both named for the position of the first double bond in the carbon chain.

- CH_3-$(CH_2)_{16}$-COOH (**stearic acid**)
- CH_3-$(CH_2)_7$-CH=CH-$(CH_2)_7$-COOH (**oleic acid**)
- 4 CH_3-$(CH_2)_4$-CH=CH-CH_2-CH=CH-$(CH_2)_7$-COOH (**linoleic acid**)
- 4 CH_3-CH_2-CH=CH-CH_2-CH=CH-CH_2-
- CH=CH-$(CH_2)_7$-COOH (**linolenic acid**)

Our bodies must obtain these two polyunsaturated acids, also called essential fatty acids, from our food. Linoleic acid is found in grains, soybeans and vegetable oils. Linolenic acid is found in leafy green vegetables and in vegetable oils. Eicosapentaenoic acid (20 carbon atoms, 5 double bonds) and docosahexaenoic acid (22 carbon atoms, 6 double bonds) are even longer-chain unsaturated omega-3 fatty acids. They are mainly found in fatty marine fish and can be produced from linoleic acid to a limited extent by the human body.

According to data from large-scale studies, omega-3 fatty acids reduce the risk of age-related macular degeneration (AMD) (Chong et al. 2009, Christen et al. 2011), but do not reduce the risk of further progression to advanced AMD in persons with pre-existing conditions (Chew 2013). Furthermore, findings suggest that omega-3 fatty acids may protect against cellular aging (Farzaneh-Far et al. 2010). It is known that abundant fish consumption naturally slows down the shortening of leukocyte telomeres (▶ Chapter 47).

One important effect of polyunsaturated omega-3 fatty acids, which are part of any varied diet, is protection against the fatal complications of coronary heart disease (Roncaglioni et al. 2013). Furthermore, the various unsaturated fatty acids are the basic building blocks for the production of **prostaglandins** (tissue hormones) that affect both vessel size and inflammatory processes. These hormones also promote the formation of leukotrienes, which have an inflammatory and hyperalgesic (pain-enhancing) effect. Finally, they play an important role in thromboxane synthesis within platelets. **Thromboxane** promotes platelet aggregation and clotting in response to injuries. Under unfavorable circumstances, however, it promotes thrombosis as well. One physiologic antagonist of thromboxane is **prostacyclin**, a prostaglandin synthesized by endothelial cells (▶ Chapter 51). For optimal synthesis of these cell messengers, the ratio of **omega-6 to omega-3 fatty acids** in our food should be approximately **5 to 1**. In Germans, for instance, this ratio is unfortunately around 20 to 1.

16 Trans-fatty acids

Not all fats are suitable for high frying at temperatures of 130–180 °C. Water in fats, like in butter, evaporates at 100 °C and then starts to spatter. Excipients from the pulp of cold-pressed oils can become altered and develop an unpleasant odor or taste when heated above 150 °C. That means good cooking fats contain little water, are free of odorants and flavorings and have a high smoke point. Examples of these include clarified butter, palm oil and refined rapeseed oil.

When certain cooking methods are used, reactions with oxygen cause nutrients high in polyunsaturated fatty acids to lose their valuable properties because oxidation breaks down the double bonds into single bonds. The health-related benefit of raw or poached fish is therefore greater than when the fish is prepared by baking, broiling or frying (► Chapter 31 and ► Chapter 32).

Another effect of high frying temperatures is that, for a split second, the double bonds are broken and small-scale rearrangements of the natural **cis-fatty acids** can take place, turning them into harmful **trans-fatty acids** (TFA). TFA elevate the levels of bad **Low-Density Lipoprotein** (LDL) cholesterol and lower those of good **High-Density Lipoprotein** (HDL) cholesterol (Dietz et Scanlon 2012). That is how TFA increase the risk for cardiovascular disease (Brouwer et al. 2013). Furthermore,

TFA can induce endothelial dysfunction (► Chapter 51), are involved in the development of insulin resistance (► Chapter 40) and increase visceral adiposity (Micha et Mozaffarian 2009). There is also an apparent connection between their intake and an increased incidence of depression (Sanchez-Villegas et al. 2011). Dietary TFA should therefore be limited to a maximum of 1 % of a person's total energy intake, i.e. approximately 2–3 g per day are considered safe. TFA are mainly found in fatty baked goods, chips, fries, dried soups, ready-made meals, candy and most brands of margarine. The amount varies by method of preparation. TFA are also produced naturally by microorganisms in the rumen of ruminant animals. That is why TFA make up 3–5 % of the total fat content of milk and beef fat.

□ **Fig. 16.1** cis-trans isomerism

17 Cholesterol

Cholesterol is a precursor for the production of vitamin D3 in the skin and of bile acids and steroid hormones in the liver. Like fatty acids, it is an essential component of cell membranes. About two-thirds of cholesterol is produced in the liver, and the remaining one-third comes from the food we eat. Genetic factors play an important role in the regulation of cholesterol levels. More than 120 gene loci of biological and clinical relevance in this context have become known to date (Blattmann et al. 2013).

The **acetic acid molecule** resulting from fat metabolism is the starting material for cell synthesis. The more saturated fatty acids stem from dietary sources, the more activated acetic acid is available to accelerate the biosynthesis of cholesterol. Moreover, high triglyceride levels are associated with correspondingly large amounts of transport proteins such as very low-density (VLD) lipoproteins. However, once these proteins have fulfilled their function after triglyceride replacement in the tissue, they can take over cholesterol from the "good" HDL transporter and subsequently transform themselves into "bad" LDL cholesterol. Through this mechanism, high triglyceride levels contribute to an increase in concentrations of harmful LDL cholesterol at the expense of the protective HDL cholesterol.

Unlike saturated fatty acids, unsaturated fatty acids (▶ Chapter 15) lower LDL-C concentrations (Sabate et al. 2011), while promoting the production of HDL cholesterol along with the activity of its receptors. These receptors are located on the surfaces of liver cells, and on cells of steroid hormone-producing organs. Unsaturated fatty acids thus positively influence cholesterol transport away from peripheral vasculature towards more central locations in the body. There is evidence suggesting that high HDL cholesterol levels are also associated with a lower risk of incident cancer (Jafri et al. 2010, Aleksandrova et al. 2014).

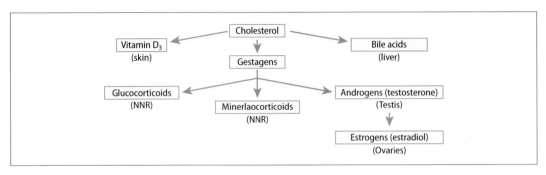

☐ **Fig. 17.1** Cholesterol as basic substance for important bioactive connections

18 Cholesterol and arteriosclerosis

The **endothelium,** the layer of cells lining the interior of blood vessels, forms a complicated interface that uses signals carried by the circulating blood to modulate vascular tone, the concentration of inflammatory cells and the coagulation cascade. Factors causing the endothelium to malfunction are high levels of **LDL** cholesterol, which in turn increase the associated risk for atherosclerosis. When macrophages attempt to remove this **LDL** cholesterol from the vascular lesions by oxidative digestion, highly reactive oxygen compounds are continuously released. These high-energy radicals inactivate the **nitric oxide** produced by the endothelium and important for normal vascular function (▶ Chapter 51). A further classification of LDL particle diameters by size reveals that it is mostly the very small and very large particles that pose the greatest risk (Grammer et al. 2014).

The molecules of the **HDL** fraction, likewise consisting of many subgroups, transport building blocks for the synthesis of nitric oxide along with messenger substances that reduce inflammatory reactions. Among others, one very important task of these **HDL** particles also consists of removing harmful cholesterol from the circulation in a process called reverse cholesterol transport to the liver (▶ Chapter 17). During this process, they are able to accept cholesterol breakdown products from the macrophages working in the arterial wall. The more effective this efflux process runs, the lower is the probability of coronary artery disease, independently of the level of HDL cholesterol (Khera et al. 2011).

Too high levels of **total cholesterol** require treatment. However, this no longer applies globally to only moderately elevated levels, as these are not generally a health risk. In 2013, this finding gave reason to correct the previous recommendation by cardiologists that cholesterol levels elevated above 200 mg/dL should strictly be regarded as requiring treatment (Stone et al. 2014, Lloyd-Jones et al. 2014). Now, cholesterol-lowering interventions are only indicated in patients with cardiovascular disease and diabetes or in individuals with a statistically elevated risk for myocardial infarction or stroke as well as for those with markedly elevated LDL cholesterol levels > 190 mg/dL.

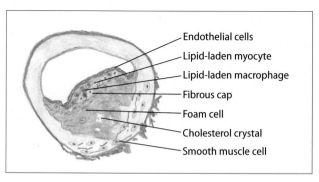

Endothelial cells
Lipid-laden myocyte
Lipid-laden macrophage
Fibrous cap
Foam cell
Cholesterol crystal
Smooth muscle cell

◻ **Fig. 18.1** Vasoconstriction in arteriosclerosis

19 Cholesterol and Alzheimer's disease

High cholesterol levels also promote the onset of Alzheimer's disease – the world's most common form of dementia. In Germany, approx. 900,000 of the nearly 1.5 million dementia sufferers have Alzheimer's, which the WHO cites as contributing to 60–70 % of dementia cases worldwide. Besides non-functioning tau proteins in the neurofibrillary bundles, other causes of Alzheimer's come from depositions (plaques) of amyloid-beta, a peptide of 42 amino acids in length (**Aβ-42**), which is found mainly in the limbic system, neocortex and hippocampus (Bateman et al. 2012). One function of the hippocampus is converting important information from short-term to long-term memory (▶ Chapter 92). The Aβ-42 peptide is formed by cleavage of a membrane-bound amyloid precursor protein in the presence of the enzyme **gamma-secretase**. The gamma-secretase-activating protein increases the activity of gamma-secretase (He et al. 2010), but so does cholesterol – with the result that elevated cholesterol levels are often accompanied by increased **amyloid plaque formation**.

Cleavage of the precursor protein also releases **Aβ-40**, a peptide two amino acids shorter than Aβ-42. This building block plays a positive role in pathogenesis insofar as it throttles **cholesterol biosynthesis** and thus also indirectly reduces the concentration of neurotoxic Aβ-42 by decreasing gamma-secretase activity. When cholesterol levels are normal, both feedback loops are in equilibrium.

When cholesterol levels are high, however, the protective function gained by lowering Aβ-40 cholesterol is often no longer effective enough, and the harmful properties of Aβ-42 predominate. This is even more relevant considering that Aβ-42 activates gamma secretase, thereby promoting further cleavage of the pre-amyloid. Aβ-42 achieves this indirectly by hindering neurons in the brain from forming **sphingomyelin**. In fact, sphingomyelin is capable of inhibiting gamma-secretase by itself. However, it can only limit pre-amyloid cleavage when it is present in sufficient concentrations.

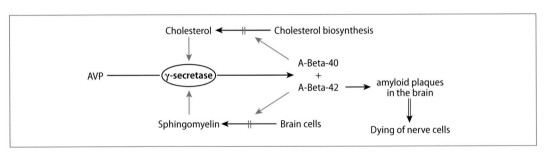

◻ **Fig. 19.1** Amyloid plaques formation: *black arrow* formation, *green arrow* activation, *red arrow* inhibition, *APP* amyloid precursor protein, *A-Beta-40* and *-42* APP splice products

20 Lipoprotein(a)

Produced in the liver, lipoprotein(a) is composed of an LDL molecule bound to apolipoprotein(a) via a disulfide bond link. Structurally, this protein component is extraordinarily homologous to the clot-dissolving plasminogen, but without being able to exercise this important function itself. On the contrary, by means of competitive inhibition, lipoprotein(a) causes the opposite: It diminishes the body's capability to dissolve any blood clots potentially formed in the vessels. Therefore, lipoprotein(a), abbreviated Lp(a), is considered an independent risk factor for the development of atherosclerosis (Kamstrup et al. 2013). Lp(a) is present in more than 30 genetic isoforms. Its genetic makeup also determines the extent of its synthesis. Approximately one-third of the population has serum Lp(a) levels above the normal range.

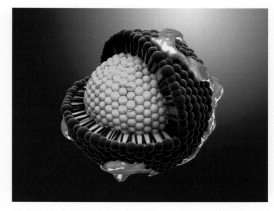

◘ **Fig. 20.1** Lipoprotein. (© Sebastian Schreiter/Springer Verlag GmbH)

There is still a widespread lack of clarity about the physiological functions of Lp(a). Epidemiological studies have shown that elevated Lp(a) levels in the blood can potentiate the negative effects of even minor increases in LDL cholesterol. Apparently, only men, but not women, are affected by this risk. And among the differently sized Lp(a) molecules, the small molecules carry an especially high risk.

Elevated Lp(a) levels are astonishingly resistant to drugs and diets. Similarly, there are no positive reactions achieved by regular exercise. Quite the opposite, endurance athletes tend to have higher levels. That is why it is assumed that Lp(a) not only has clearly atherogenic properties, but also that it plays a role in the processes involved in repairing the microtrauma to the tissue constantly accompanying physical exercise. This presumption is supported by the fact that Lp(a) is also considered a moderate acute-phase protein (► Chapter 61). During inflammatory diseases, increases of 2 to 3 times the normal levels have been described.

21 Minerals

Minerals are neither produced nor metabolized in our body. They are eliminated via various mechanisms and have to be constantly resupplied with our food intake.

Sodium, potassium, chloride and **phosphate** are abundant in the foods we eat. The daily requirement, for example, for sodium chloride is 2–3 g. The WHO recommends consuming no more than 5 grams of salt per day. In fact, we regularly consume quite a bit more than this in the form of table salt. According to studies conducted by the Centers for Disease Control and Prevention in Georgia (USA), most of this amount is hidden in ready-made meals and restaurant dishes. Even bread contains a lot of salt. The EU Commission recommends a policy to keep the salt content at 1 % of the volume of flour. Bakers in Germany, for example, use about twice this amount. Indeed, too-high salt intake can be harmful because it frequently leads to high blood pressure (▶ Chapter 53) and, consequently, to a greater incidence of myocardial infarctions, strokes and chronic heart diseases (Strazzullo et al. 2009, Bibbins-Domingo et al. 2010, Cobb et al. 2014). Around 30 % of people with normal blood pressure and about half of hypertension sufferers prove to be salt-sensitive at the time of diagnosis. It is these individuals in particular who benefit from a low-salt diet. According to a meta-analysis of 107 randomized interventions, around 1.65 million deaths could be avoided annually worldwide by limiting salt consumption to a maximum of 5 g per day (Mozaffarian et al. 2014).

Our daily potassium requirement of 3.5 g (WHO recommendation) can be easily met by eating grains, vegetables, bananas or nuts. The results of large-scale cohort studies with long observation periods have demonstrated that a potassium-rich diet significantly reduces the risk of stroke (D'Elia et al. 2011, Aburto et al. 2013). Milk, meat, fish and vegetables provide the necessary 0.7 g of phosphate (German Association for Nutrition). Too much phosphate can be harmful to the kidneys and blood vessels. The readily absorbable phosphate additives in many foods are the problem (Ritz et al. 2012).

Calcium is found in dairy products, vegetables and certain mineral waters. It is important for bone metabolism, signal transmission across synapses and triggering muscle contractions. Calcium is also a cofactor in blood coagulation. Long-term excess calcium intake of 1500 mg or more increases the risk of cardiovascular mortality (Xiao et al. 2013, Michaelsson et al. 2013).

> A daily intake of 1000 mg calcium and 300–400 mg of magnesium is desirable.

Magnesium is a component of the activity centers of many enzymes and is involved in about 300 different metabolic processes. It lowers vascular tone and muscle contraction. High magnesium intake is associated with a lower risk of type 2 diabetes (Schulze et al. 2007, Kim et al. 2010, Dong et al. 2011, Hruby et al. 2014). Magnesium deficiency can lead to muscle cramps, increases in blood pressure and arrhythmic cardiac death (Chiuve et al. 2013). Only around 1 % of total magnesium is found in the blood plasma. Roughly 60 % is present in the bones and 35 % in muscle tissue. The rest is distributed in the liver and other bodily fluids. Major sources of magnesium include whole grain products, nuts and most types of fruits and vegetables.

22 Trace elements

Minerals with a daily requirement of less than 100 mg are called trace elements (Tab. 22.1). **Iron** is one of them. In the hemoglobin molecule, iron is crucial for oxygen transport. Men have about 50 mg of iron per kg of body weight, while women have around 40 mg. Meat, fish and legumes are all important sources of iron.

About 2–4 g of **Zinc** is present in the human body and can be found in various tissues. It is a component of some enzymes, like lactate dehydrogenase. Zinc deficiency causes wound healing disorders, skin diseases, hair loss and impairment of the immune defenses. Sources of Zinc include meat, milk, seafood and wheat germ.

Chromium participates in insulin's function and **cobalt** is critical for the mechanism of action of vitamin B_{12}. Cobalt also plays an important role in the formation of red blood cells and for the activation of several enzymes. **Copper** is essential for collagen synthesis and the hormones adrenaline and noradrenaline. **Manganese** facilitates bone development and is involved in coagulation. **Molybdenum** is vital to uric acid metabolism and the detoxification of alcohol. Deficiency symptoms are rare for these 5 trace elements. They can be found in whole grain products, nuts, milk, yeast and fungi. **Silicon** is primarily found in fruits and vegetables and is important for the structure and function of connective tissue.

Selenium's meaning for health is very versatile. It is a crucial component of the active groups of about 35 different selenoproteins. Selenium is essential for specific immunity and normal thyroid function, and provides a protective effect against cardiovascular diseases. It is found in cereals, seafood and Brazil nuts. Selenium deficiency is also rare.

Iodine belongs to the functional group of the thyroid hormones T_3 and T_4. Iodized table salt and seafood are both important sources of iodine. **Fluoride** promotes tooth formation and healthy bone structure. Egg yolk, milk and seafood contain abundant amounts of fluoride.

 Tab. 22.1 Daily need for trace elements

Micronutrient	Daily need (adults)
Chrome	30–100 µg
Iron	10–15 mg
Fluoride	3.1–3.8 mg
iodine	180–200 µg
Cobalt	2 µg
Copper	1–1.5 mg
Manganese	2–5 mg
Molybdenum	50–100 µg
Selenium	30–70 µg
Silicon	30 mg
Zinc	7–10 mg

23 Vitamins

An individual's daily vitamin requirement depends on their level of physical activity, age, diet composition and any existing pregnancy or diseases (◻ Tab. 23.1). The body can store fat-soluble vitamins. Vitamin D represents a special case, as its character is more similar to that of a hormone. Vitamin K occurs in the three forms K_1, K_2 and K_3. Only the variants K_1 and K_2 are important for our body's metabolism.

With today's oversupply of food, vitamin deficiencies are now rare. Despite this fact, the benefits of vitamin supplementation have been studied extensively (Neuhouser et al. 2009, Blencowe et al. 2010, Clarke et al. 2010, Bestwick et al. 2014). The conferral of any benefit has only been proven for the vitamin D3 hormone (▶ Chapter 24) and, to a certain extent, for folate as well.

Large-scale studies and meta-analyses with more than 100,000 participants each and study periods of several years have produced rather negative results on the additional intake of other vitamins (Schürks et al. 2010, Mursu et al. 2011). The risk of death in populations taking certain vitamin supplements, e.g. the combination of the vitamins A, C and E (but also vitamin E supplementation in isolation) is slightly elevated.

However, the suspicion that high-dose treatment with vitamin A would reduce bone density, thereby increasing the risk of fractures, has not been confirmed in large-scale studies (Vestergaard et al. 2010, Ambrosini et al. 2013).

◻ **Tab. 23.1** Daily need for vitamins

Vitamins	Daily need
Water-soluble	
B1 (Thiamine)	1.0–1.3 mg
B2 (Riboflavin)	1.2–1.5 mg
B3 (Nicotinic)	13–17 mg
B5 (Pantothenic)	6 mg
B6 (Pyridoxine)	1.2–1.5 mg
B12 (Cobalamin)	3.0 µg
C	100 mg
Folate	300 µg
H (Biotin)	30–60 µg
Fat-soluble	
A	0.8–1.0 mg
D	20–50 µg
E	12–15 mg
K	60–80 µg

Daily intake of 550 µg of folate for 5 weeks before conception and during the first 12 weeks after the inception of pregnancy significantly reduces the risk of neural tube defects.

24 The vitamin D3 hormone

Most tissue types carry receptors for the vitamin D_3 hormone and are therefore receptive to its myriad control signals. It exercises a regulatory function over the activity of at least 200 genes. One important responsibility of this hormone lies in **bone metabolism** (▶ Chapter 75) and in **optimizing the body's neuromuscular coordination**. Because 1.25-dihydroxyvitamin D3 is coupled to special nucleus receptors, it inhibits elevated cell division rates and promotes cell differentiation. Therefore, vitamin D is also presumed to play a decisive role in reducing the risk for many chronic diseases. For example, numerous studies have repeatedly described the relationship between sufficiently high vitamin D_3 levels and a lower risk of various types of cancer (Peterlik et al. 2009, Jenab et al. 2010, Schöttker et al. 2013). In the presence of high vitamin D_3 levels, moreover, the risk for diabetes is halved, blood pressure tends to be normal and the risk for cardiovascular diseases is markedly reduced (Parker et al. 2010, Brøndum-Jacobsen et al. 2012). Under these conditions, the functions exercised by monocytes and macrophages in the immune system are optimized (▶ Chapter 61) and mental performance in the elderly is stabilized (Llewellyn et al. 2010). That said, it still remains to be proven that vitamin D actually always causes all of these effects. It might be conceivable that it is the other way around, i.e., that malignant diseases lower vitamin D levels, i.e. the low levels are thus a sequela of malignant tumors and not their cause (Autier et al. 2014). The results of the VITAL study investigating the causality of the effects of Vitamin D are not anticipated to be presented until the year 2017.

The daily recommended intake of vitamin D_3 is 20–50 μg = 800–2000 IU. Only a diet consisting of the abundant consumption of fatty marine fish and milk products as well as 30 minutes of sunlight to the head and lower arms during the summer months from April to September guarantee the intake of sufficient levels. As the skin gets tanner, its vitamin D synthesis diminishes. Similarly, the elderly produce less than younger people. And the higher the air pollution, the lower is the necessary proportion of UV-B (280–315 nm) absorbed from sunlight.

The hurdle for sufficient vitamin D supply is high, making non-diagnosed deficiencies a frequent occurrence. 25-dihydroxyvitamin D_3 is a basic measure of vitamin D status. the desirable range for **serum levels** are **30–70 μg/l**. According to data from the Robert Koch Institute in Germany, only approximately 40 % of adults and 15 % of 3- to 17-year-old children have levels within this range. In rare cases, chronic high-dose intake of the vitamin can induce vitamin D intoxication accompanied by a rise in blood calcium concentrations, subsequently leading to calcification of tendons, ligaments, joints, vessels and internal organs.

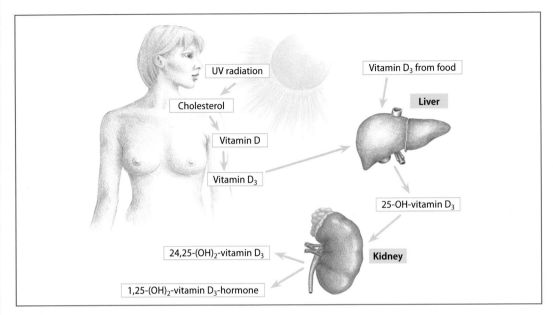

■ Fig. 24.1 Production of active vitamin D3 hormone

25 Secondary plant compounds

Besides the commonly known main ingredients, our nutrients and luxury foods often contain many other bioactive compounds (◻ Tab. 25.1). The number of individual compounds is estimated in the range of 60,000 – 100,000. The phytochemicals present in the various types of fruits and vegetables have formed over the millennia of evolution to protect plants against UV radiation, pests and dysregulation during their growth.

Secondary plant compounds only occur in trace amounts and are mostly localized in peels and seeds. They are not temperature-sensitive and therefore made more digestible by boiling or cooking. Since ancient times, people have lived on a regular diet consisting of a broad spectrum of such bioactive plant compounds and thereby optimized their nutritional intake. In a mixed diet, secondary plant compounds, around 10,000 of which we consume regularly, make up approximately 1.5 g of our daily nutrition.

Examples of these important nutrients include the flavonoids in general and the **flavanols** in particular, which belong to one of 9 flavonoid subgroups. Some flavanols of note include the antioxidants epicatechin and epigallocatechin gallate. Both occur in tea, cocoa and in many types of fruit. Flavanols are inversely associated with incident type 2 diabetes (Zamora-Ros et al. 2014), they slow down arteriosclerotic processes by limiting the range of motion of smooth muscle cells within the vessel wall, inhibit platelet function and lower blood pressure by blocking the formation of endothelin, a potent vasoconstrictor. The **anthocyanidins**, another subgroup of the flavonoids, also have an antihypertensive action. They give pigment to the blue, purple and red fruits. Their positive effect on blood pressure was shown in a 14-year prospective study on 156,962 participating women and men (Cassidy et al. 2011).

Despite the rapidly growing body of knowledge on a diverse range of plant compounds, which usually only release their health-promoting properties in complex mixtures, they have not been administered for the targeted treatment of specific diseases thus far. During certain drug-based interventions, it is important for patients to avoid furanocoumarin derivatives present in grapefruit because interactions with their breakdown products can change the bioavailability of over 80 drugs in the body (Bailey et al. 2013, Pirmohamed 2013).

◻ **Tab. 25.1** Important secondary plant substances

Substance group	Main effects
Carotinoids	1, 3, 6, 8
Glucosinolates	1, 2, 6
Monoterpenes	1, 2
Phytosterols	1, 6
Protease inhibitors	1, 3
Saponins	1, 2, 6, 7, 8
Sulfides	1, 2, 3, 4, 5, 6, 7, 8
Flavonoids	1, 2, 3, 4, 5, 6, 7, 8
Phenolic acids	1, 2, 3
Phytoestrogens	1, 3

1 antitumor, *2* antibiotic, *3* antioxidant, *4* anticoagulant, *5* blood pressure regulating, *6* cholesterol-lowering, *7* anti-inflammatory, *8* immuno-stimulating

26 Dietary fiber

Dietary fiber is primarily found in fruits, vegetables, grains and legumes. For humans, they are indigestible. Nevertheless, their high fiber content is indispensable for normal bowel motility. By absorbing water, the fibers swell and thereby stimulate peristalsis. By promoting peristalsis, the time that any toxins are in contact with the intestinal wall is shortened. Moreover, dietary fiber binds cholesterol and bile acids and positively influences the bacterial flora in our gut.

According to data from the EPIC study, a diet consisting of an abundance of fruits and vegetables lowers the risk for cardiovascular diseases (Crowe et al. 2011). And a diet rich in fiber (especially one consisting of wholegrain products) also prevents type 2 diabetes (Schulze et al. 2007). 17 g of dietary fiber from whole grains reduce the risk for diabetes by one-third compared to a daily consumption of only 7 g. A more recent evaluation of this study confirms the positive effect of dietary fiber (Sluijs et al. 2010), as do the results of the Nurses' Health Study on nearly 200,000 participants (Sun et al. 2010) and the results of an analysis of prospective cohort studies on 488,293 participants (Yao et al. 2014). Plenty of dietary fiber should therefore help prolong life. Exactly this in fact is the result of the NIH-AARP Diet and Health Study, which observed 388,122 participants from this perspective over a period of 9 years (Park et al. 2011).

Even the portion of dietary fiber, especially deriving from the consumption of fruit and vegetables alone, is associated with a lower risk of death from

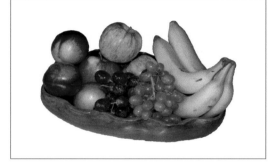

◻ Fig. 26.1

cardiovascular diseases and cancer (Leenders et al. 2013, Oyebode et al. 2014, Wang et al. 2014). The higher the consumption, the greater is the protective effect. In this regard, vegetables obviously have a stronger effect than fruit, and raw vegetables have a stronger effect than cooked vegetables.

Cellulose, pectin, lignin and similar structural components are only found in plant-based foodstuffs.

Dietary fiber cannot be metabolized. Their proportion in food should amount to approx. 30g per day.

27 Antioxidants

Combustion processes are an indispensable requirement for organisms to generate energy. So-called **"reactive oxygen species" (ROS)** are generated by these processes, but also arise from environmental toxins, cigarette smoke and pharmaceutical drugs. The reactive oxygen species are present as radicals, a state in which they possess an extremely high energy potential.

Free radicals perform meaningful physiological tasks. Formed by leukocytes during immune defenses, they destroy bacteria, for example (▶ Chapter 61). They also fulfill an important protective function in the blood vessels in the form of nitrogen monoxide (NO) (▶ Chapter 51). Unfortunately, their most common reactions often also cause destructive effects on cells and tissue. These reactions are presumed to be involved in the development of cardiovascular diseases or cancer and also potentially accelerate the aging process.

However, many enzymes, metabolic products and ingredients in our food have an antioxidant action. A sensible diet rich in vitamins and secondary plant compounds is therefore the best protection against excessive radical production. The amount of antioxidants is particularly high in organically grown fruit and vegetables (Baranski et al. 2014).

Possible therapies with and/or the preventive use of antioxidants are constantly being propagated. However, the results of all studies available to date have not shown that any positive effects are conferred.

Superoxide dismutase is one example from the well-functioning arsenal of endogenous free radical scavengers. Together with **catalase**, an oxidoreductase enzyme, they use hydrogen peroxide to convert oxygen radicals to water and oxygen. The increased combustion processes during physical activity facilitate these endogenous repair systems. The multiple radicals produced here apparently have a long-term effect like a vaccine against oxidative stress. There is, however, evidence that frequent drug intake with larger amounts of vitamins C and E can suppress the health-promoting antioxidant effect of physical exercise (Ristow et al. 2009).

Important biological antioxidants include: β-Carotin, coeruloplasmin, a large variety of secondary plant compounds, glutathione, glutathione peroxidase, haptoglobin, catalase, superoxide dismutase, transferrin, vitamins C and E.

28 Influence of diet on immunity

Constantly and in huge quantities, we assimilate minutely small particles from the microcosm surrounding us when we breathe, eat food or have bodily contact, but are only able to detect such traces to a very limited extent. for instance – thanks to our sense of smell and taste – in rotten food. This particulate matter, also referred to as antigens, however, poses a permanent threat to our health and our lives because the particles can disrupt the delicate balance between the physiological and biochemical reactions in the body in myriad ways. That is why immune mechanisms that work independently are needed to control these reactions. They are organized in our immune system. Because antigens can penetrate or occur at any random site in the body, the around 2 trillion immune cells are distributed throughout the entire organism. Approximately 1 % of these cells are on constant patrol within our body. The circulation velocity required for a single passage through all organs is amazingly quick at 30 minutes. That way, they can control the immune defenses in every body structure and eliminate everything they identify as foreign. Thus, our immune system very decisively dictates the degree of our well-being and of our consummate health, ranging from the common cold to life-threatening diseases.

Our diet is eminently important when it comes to attaining optimum immunity (see also ► Chapter 61 to ► Chapter 63). For instance, overeating tends to lower both the number as well as the activities of T lymphocytes and natural killer cells (NK cells), limiting antibody synthesis. High concentrations of LDL cholesterol can change the lipid composition of cell membranes, thereby impairing lymphocyte signal transmissions. Under-eating, linked to protein deficiency as well as deficits in vitamins and minerals, diminishes the function of the secondary lymphatic organs and leads to reduced lymphocyte counts. Cytokine formation, particularly that of IFNγ (interferon γ), IL-1 and IL-2 (interleukin 1 and 2), is impaired, the concentrations of complement fractions are lowered and the mobility of neutrophilic granulocytes reduced.

Although most nutritional deficiencies in industrialized nations are usually only encountered in elderly persons, when they do occur, they exacerbate even further any incipient immune deficiency that becomes manifest. Among others, they are based on the fact that, in old age, stem cell production in the bone marrow slows down, immunocompetent cells undergo less active cell division (as a result of a previously impaired IL-2 synthesis) and acute-phase reactions become interference-prone.

A balanced diet and the maintenance of normal body weight and lipid metabolism will strengthen the immune system.

As free radical scavengers, vitamins C and E support the immune defenses, while vitamins A, C and B_6 additionally enhance the activity of immune cells. Supplemental vitamin preparations are not required for this. The trace element selenium is important for phagocytosis as well as for the cytotoxic activity of CD8+ lymphocytes and NK cells. Sufficient iron levels have a positive effect on the number of B lymphocytes, on antibody production and on concentrations of C3 and C4 complement fractions. Iron, moreover, facilitates phagocytosis and T-cell response.

Another important trace element in this context is zinc. Its deficiency impairs the functions of NK cells and CD4+ helper cells as well as the mechanisms of antigen presentation. Lycopene, the carotenoid pigment that makes tomatoes red, improves the cell division capability of lymphocytes and leads to increased IL-2 synthesis.

29 Functional foods

"Let food be thy medicine
and medicine be thy food."

This quote, attributed to Hippocrates, reflects the age-old desire of people to heal or even prevent diseases with certain foods. The term "functional food," coined in Japan and the USA in the 1970s, refers to foodstuffs fortified with different probiotics or microorganisms, the specific health-promoting benefits of which must be sufficiently scientifically substantiated. Thanks to the constantly rising health awareness among the population, functional foods are gaining in popularity. Examples of popular products include types of margarine enriched with phytosterols that block the absorption of cholesterol from the gut and can thereby lower LDL cholesterol levels in the blood or probiotic milk products containing highly resistant lactic acid bacteria intended to strengthen the immune system and improve the intestinal flora. The addition of calcium to fruit juice, eggs with a very high content of unsaturated fatty acids, bread with linolenic acid or the general enrichment of foods with various vitamins constitute further examples.

More recent trends on the foods market include genetically modified products, e. g. tomatoes with double the content of the red carotenoid pigment lycopene, green lettuce with more xanthophyll (lutein) or iron-enriched types of rice. Meanwhile, functional foods are more commonly being re-ferred to as nutraceuticals or designer foods, and naturally are not designed to help acute symptoms. rather,

> they mitigate the long-term health risks from cancer, cardiovascular diseases or chronic degenerative conditions and slow down aging processes.

That said, the effects of functional food targeting the long term are exactly what makes it difficult to assess their benefits. Potential side effects like in the above-mentioned types of margarine leak out to the public very slowly and skepticism is advised because plant-based foods contain hundreds of substances that do not exert the positive effects attributed to them until combined together. It is therefore no wonder that there has been a lack of scientific substantiation of the postulated benefits of functional foods by large-scale studies to date. Likewise, answers still need to be found to questions about changes in taste, the optimization of composition and particularly about any adverse health effects (Crowe et Francis 2013). Functional food products are way more expensive than normal produce. The German Nutrition Society has justifiably issued statements that nutritional defects cannot be compensated for with functional food.

30 Chemicals in plant-based foodstuffs

Our current agriculture industry has become insep-
arable from **pesticides**. In Germany alone, over
35,000 tons are used annually. These include 250
approved active agents in approx. 1,900 products.
on the European level, nearly 800 active agents are
used in around 20,000 products (◻ Tab. 30.1). Her-
bicides and fungicides are used most frequently. The
widespread use of sprayed chemicals over the years
has continually burdened our soil and groundwater
with ever larger amounts of pollutants.

Their acute effects on the body have meanwhile
been well researched given that even cautious estimates in the developing countries state that over
200,000 people die annually from exposure to
chemicals (Prüss-Ustün et al. 2011). By and large,
however, most consumers lack true knowledge
about the chronic effects of pesticides. An increase
in the rates of cancer and allergies is discussed, as
are other disorders of the immune system. Pesticides can affect human fertility and pose risks to

◻ **Tab. 30.1** Classification of pesticides by target organism

Pesticide	Against
Fungicides	Fungi
Herbicides	Weeds
Insecticides	Insects
Molluscicides	Snails, slugs
Nematicides	Nematodes

the development of the unborn child. By impairing
the nervous system, insecticides appear to lead to a
higher frequency of dementia syndromes in elderly
farmers. It is **fungicides** and **insecticides** that harbor
the greatest risks for humans.

Thoroughly washing fruit and vegetables under
running water can remove a portion of the pollutant
residues, although it is better to peel this kind of
produce. Plant-based foods should be bought when
they are in season where they grow indigenously.
Pesticide exposure is then the lowest. Plant compounds from foreign countries usually have a higher burden with pesticide residues, while organically
grown crops always contain less (Baranski et al.
2014).

> The pesticide residue limit on food of 10 μg/kg
> should not be exceeded.

◻ **Fig. 30.1** EU bio logo since July 1, 2010

31 Health risks from heating foods I

Our standard foods can be burdened with toxins from their multiple processing stages. Pesticides, aflatoxins from molds, solanine in the green spots on tomatoes, antibiotics administered to livestock or dioxins in meat and eggs are further examples of repeated food issues triggering concern by the public. Apparently, the discussions about a health-conscious diet have given less attention to the toxins that can be formed, for example, by the way we prepare our meals during the heating of certain foods.

The **polycyclic aromatic hydrocarbons (PAHs)** have long been an issue in this connection. One typical representative of this drug class is **benzo(a) pyrene**, a compound deriving from the highly toxic benzene and a potent carcinogen. Benzo(a)pyrene occurs as a product of many incomplete combustion processes and is also present, among others, in cigarette smoke (► Chapter 93) and in automotive exhaust fumes. When such compounds develop in smokers or particularly when grilling over charcoal that is not thoroughly glowing, they can precipitate on the grilled meat and build up. Melting fat and fat droppings on the coals facilitate the formation of PAHs. Therefore, important protection interventions like a grill with a lateral arrangement and wrapping the food to be grilled in aluminum foil should be used.

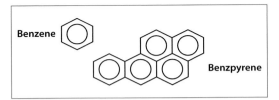

□ Fig. 31.1

Heterocyclic aromatic amines (HAA) increase cancer risk (Zheng et Lee 2009). They are formed from amino acids and creatine when meat from beef, pork and fowl or fish are processed for longer periods at temperatures higher than 150 °C.

> Just to play it safe, darkly smoked and solid burned crusts should always be cut off.

Giving in to the desire to eat grilled meat along with darkly toasted bread or bread with very dark crust is tempting fate with additional health hazards. The is due to the **monochloropropanediol (3-MCPD)**, a carcinogenic substance produced from table salt and from the fat cleaved from a glycerol moiety at high heat.

32 Health risks from heating food II

It is primarily red meat (beef, pork lamb) that heating can turn into the source of several carcinogenic agents. Ranking alongside polycyclic hydrocarbons and heterocyclic aromatic amines are the **nitrosamines**. Even pathogenic viruses in the meat might be causes of cancer, as the Nobel Prize Laureate Harald zur Hausen suspected. Several studies, including the 2 analyses of the prospective NIH-AARP study (▶ Chapter 3) from the USA on over 500,000 persons aged between 50–71 years, have shown that frequent ingestion of processed and unprocessed meat from female cows increases the risk of esophageal, lung, liver and bowel cancer (Sinha et al. 2009, Cross et al. 2007, 2010, Keszei et al. 2012).

According to the results of a large meta-analysis, daily consumption of as little as 50 g of processed red meat in the form of sausages, bacon, hamburgers, kebab etc. is associated with an additional increase of around 40 % in the risk for cardiovascular diseases and approximately 19 % in the risk for type 2 diabetes (Micha et al. 2010). Data from the EPIC study prove that the risk of early death is 18 % higher in persons exhibiting this dietary behavior (Rohrmann et al. 2013). Causes attributed to this include the higher salt content and the increased number of nitrosamines produced by the heating process involved in cooking these meats. They potentially also promote the development of Alzheimer's disease. Regarding type 2 diabetes, according to data from very large long-term studies, even unprocessed red meat significantly increases the risk of disease (Pan et al. 2011, 2013).

Major speculation is linked to the question as to whether **acrylamide**, long known as a neurotoxin,

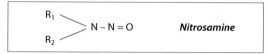

❏ Fig. 32.1

❏ Fig. 32.2

is also mutagenic and can cause cancer as well. Acrylamide and its similarly very harmful, oxidative metabolite **glycidamide** are formed from the heating process of anhydrous, starch- or sugar-containing foods with the amino acid asparagine.

> Acrylamide exposure is particularly high in French fries, potato chips and home fries.

This asparagine occurs in dietary proteins. Having said that, humans have been consuming heated food for thousands of years – which is how long acrylamide has been present in our food. That is why the recommendations for lowering any actual or presumed risk currently only refer to the temperatures applied. For example, baking temperatures should not exceed 190 °C (or 170 °C in convection ovens) and frying temperatures should not exceed 160 °C. When the food becomes golden brown within the shortest possible baking or frying time, then this has the utmost priority over browning them too dark.

33 Health risks from flavor enhancers?

The manufacturers of store-bought convenience meals regularly add a plethora of chemicals like preservatives, food colorings, emulgators, stabilizers, thickening agents as well as flavor enhancers. In the European Union, approx. 320 different food additives are currently approved.

> Approximately half of all raw food materials contain such additives.

The permissible amounts are measured to prevent health damage over a lifetime. Nevertheless, the acceptable daily intake (ADI) values on which these limits are based only apply to adults. No values have been set for children.

The flavor enhancers frequently used are highly controversial. For example, monosodium glutamate has been linked to the development of Alzheimer's disease, Parkinson's disease and the Chinese restaurant syndrome (headache, nausea, numbness in the neck, tightness in the thorax and burning skin) among others. Given that the body of scientific data, however, is highly inadequate, neither the national professional societies nor international institutions like the WHO have spoken out for a ban on glutamate additives.

In normal amounts, glutamate is even essential for life. Glutamate is a salt of glutamic acid which is a key component of very many endogenous proteins (▶ Chapter 4). Therefore, glutamate is also often present in the proteins of our food, as the following examples will show.

> Glutamic acid as a percentage of total protein by weight:
> Whole grain wheat flour = 32, cow's milk = 21, unpolished rice = 20, walnuts = 19, beef or chicken meat = 15, salmon = 14, egg = 13

Several types of produce like tomatoes, cheese or yeast contain larger amounts of "free" glutamate.

> Additive glutamate of up to 1 g per 100 g of our foods is permitted (Council Directive 92/2/EC). It is prohibited to add glutamate to baby food.

Even though excessive amounts of glutamate might not directly cause illness, they still obviously indirectly pose a problem by promoting obesity. Indeed, glutamate is one of several peripheral neurotransmitters that intervene in appetite regulation in the brain (▶ Chapter 12 and ▶ Chapter 14). It suppresses the saturation signals, so the individual keeps eating. But it keeps people eating more for another reason. Namely, glutamate gives even the blandest, cheapest meals a pleasant intensive flavor. This is so pronounced that it meanwhile counts as a fifth basic taste after salt, sweet, sour and bitter. It is called **umami**, which means yummy, deliciousness or a pleasant savory taste in Japanese, and was coined in 1908 by the Japanese chemist Kikunae Ikeda. Weight gains related to monosodium glutamate have been observed frequently (He et al. 2011).

34 Ethanol – small molecule, strong toxin

Alcohols are chemical hydrocarbons where a hydrogen atom is substituted by the functional hydroxyl group (-OH). Ethyl alcohol is the only form that is palatable for humans. It derives from ethane and is thus a 2-carbon compound.

In our world of today, alcoholic drinks are very prevalent. One major reason for their increased consumption is the enormous investment in advertising by the alcohol industry to promote their products. In Germany, they amounted to around € 562 million in 2012. 10.8 million citizens of the Federal Republic of Germany drink alcohol in amounts that pose a risk to their health. According to the Drug Report commissioned by German Federal Government, approximately 1.4 million people between 18 and 65 years of age and 400,000 people over 65 suffer from alcoholism. The risk of a subsequent alcohol addiction is higher the earlier adolescents start drinking alcohol. And this risk is especially high when alcohol consumption starts during puberty, because the brain is in a very critical maturation stage when the decline in cerebral blood flow begins (Satterthwaite et al. 2014).

Alcohol is a cytotoxin that when enjoyed regularly even in small amounts damages nearly all organs in the body. Via acetaldehyde, an intermediate of the biological metabolism of alcohol, it increases the risk for cancer of the oral and pharyngeal cavity, larynx, esophagus, breast, stomach, liver, pancreas and bowel (Allen et al. 2009, Schütze et al. 2011).

In addition to frequent episodes of atrial fibrillation (Kodoma et al. 2011), potential sequelae of excessive alcohol intake include: Elevated blood pressure, myocardial infarction, stroke, inflammation of the liver, pancreas, stomach and bowel, fatty liver, liver cirrhosis, diabetes and nerve cells damage

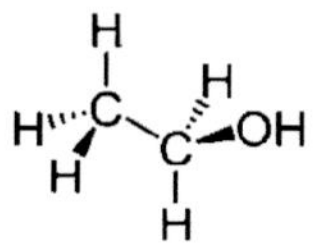

Fig. 34.1 Structural formula of alcohol

accompanied by increased irritability, depression, psychoses and young-onset dementia (Nordström et al. 2013). Life expectancy is markedly limited (Zaridze et al. 2014).

The socioeconomic damage caused by alcohol abuse is tremendous. In the year 2013, the costs in Germany were cited at € 27 billion annually. This stands in contrast with the alcohol tax levied of € 3.4 billion. Every day, approximately 40 alcohol-related fatalities occur in Germany, and 2.5 million worldwide annually according to data from the WHO. Therefore, if at all, alcohol should not be drunk every day: Women should not drink more than 10 g and men not more than 20 g of pure alcohol a day. Even moderate alcohol consumption decreases total brain volume, in females more than in males (Paul et al. 2008). The smallest amounts of alcohol are taboo for women during pregnancy - from the beginning to the end.

An intoxicated binge permanently destroys the function of millions of brain cells.

Because alcoholic fermentation occurs in fresh fruit and alcohol is similarly formed by lactic acid fermentation, even healthy produce will contain trace amounts of alcohol, albeit not harmful even to children, according to current knowledge.

35 General nutritional recommendations for healthy people

Some of the nutritional principles for healthy people include:
- A balanced, varied and low-fat diet
- It is best to use vegetable oils as fat
- Fewer meat and meat products and more fish. if meat, then preferably white over red
- Eat half a kilogram of fruit and vegetables daily
- Abundant intake of grain products
- Limit sugar consumption to 10 % of the caloric requirements at most

> The higher the products are in the food pyramid, the less frequently they should be eaten.

These general recommendations are nothing new. They were phrased similarly by our forefathers and differ only slightly from the nowadays very popular Mediterranean cuisine (Sofi et al. 2008, Fung et al. 2009). The latter place even more value on fish, the

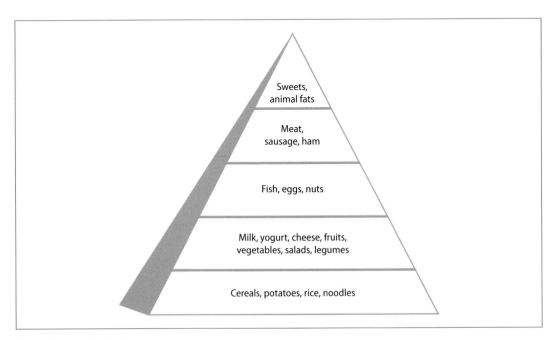

□ **Fig. 35.1** Food pyramid

abundant consumption of fruit, vegetables and nuts and replace saturated fatty acids with olive oil (Mitrou et al. 2007, Buckland et al. 2010, Kastorini et al. 2011, Crowe et al. 2013, Ruiz-Canela et al. 2014). Such a diet is also related to a lower likelihood of incident cognitive impairment (Tsivgoulis et al. 2013) and, according to data from large-scale studies, can prolong life (Bao et al. 2013, Oyebode et al. 2014).

Because lifetime eating habits are imprinted in childhood, children should learn early to follow a healthy diet. This is not easy, but still possible when the parents practice this in front of the children during regularly shared family meals (Hammons et Fiese 2011). This includes, among others, also taking enough time for breakfast in the morning (Cahill et al. 2013) and learning to endure hunger for limited periods. Children who partake of their meals regularly together with their families eat more fruit and vegetables than children without such shared meals (Christian et al. 2013).

Concerning the special problem of portion sizes, thought should be given to the fact that the mechanisms of natural satiety regulation can also diminish in the early years of life (▶ Chapter 12 to ▶ Chapter 14). Therefore, children themselves will often eat much more when more is offered to them. The consequence of this is that they will build fat cells within their genetically predisposed range. This number remains permanent when they reach adulthood. And the number of fat cells is a co-determinant factor in the magnitude of potential obesity (▶ Chapter 37).

36 Recommended fluid intake

The average human body is made up of around 60 % water. Through the skin, but also the kidneys, intestines and respirated air, it loses 1.5–2.5 liters of water daily and much more during activities in hot environments or from fever or diarrhea. The losses are compensated for by ingestion of water from solid food (500–700 ml per day) or metabolism (200–300 ml per day) and from drinking fluids. Under everyday conditions, the recommended drinking amount is approximately 20 ml per kg of body weight, and 15 ml in persons older than 65 years. This includes diuretic fluids like coffee or tea. Although caffeine contained in these drinks inhibits the sodium and water absorption in the renal tubules, regular enjoyment of caffeine is associated with a rapid habituation process and coffee or tea then affect the fluids balance according to the ingested amount of water consumed.

Even though the feeling of thirst is occasionally unreliable (particularly in older people), the common recommendation to drink copious amounts of fluids daily is questionable. Positive effects on appetite, weight, skin, renal function or on other organs have not been scientifically substantiated to date.

What is undisputed, however, is the fact that dehydration should be avoided. Even moderate water losses can cause sluggishness, fatigue and possibly even headaches as well. Fluid deficits starting at 2 % (approximately 1000 ml) can seriously impair physical and mental performance. Fluids intake of less than 800 ml per day have been associated with a limited concentration potential of the kidneys.

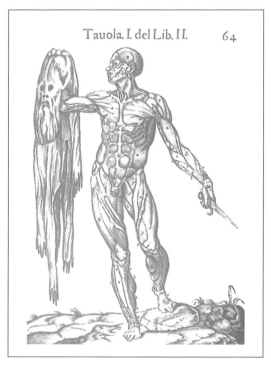

Fig. 36.1 Bercerra (1560), Anatomia del corpo humano. (Courtesy of Andreas Verlag, Salzburg)

Urea levels are then elevated and substantially cloud consciousness. The parallel elevations in increasing potassium concentrations trigger tachycardia and cardiac rhythmus disorders. Chronically high losses of bodily water are life-threatening.

37 Evolution fattens its progeny

For millions of years, our evolution has been characterized by limited nutritional resources. Nutritional deficiency was therefore constantly much more dangerous than nutritional surplus and optimal utilization of food always provided a survival benefit.

From this perspective, the XXXL people of today belong to the evolutionary elite. A claim to fame most of them would be glad to divorce themselves from. Sixty percent of Germans are overweight. As many as one-eighth of all children and adolescents are too fat. The tragic consequence of this fact is that most overweight 10- to 13-year-olds will also be too heavy as adults. Among others, they are at an increased risk for high blood pressure, developing coronary heart disease, stroke, bowel cancer and diabetes already in middle age (Bjorge et al. 2008, Adams et al. 2014, Bairdain et al. 2014). Increased body size in childhood is associated with a greater risk of diabetes in adulthood, as confirmed by analyses of the data on over 109,000 participants in Nurses' Health Study II. However, the risk normalizes when the affected women become lean again later in young adulthood (Yeung et al. 2010).

There are genetic co-factors respon-sible for overweight and obesity. They not only influence the distribution of adipose tissue (▶ Chapter 38), but are also involved in the regulation of feelings of hunger and satiation (Speliotes et al. 2010). However, the effects of genes overall is rather low, the risk for an elevated body mass index is mainly determined (to approximately 95 %) by a person's lifestyle. For hundreds and hundreds of generations, our genetic potential has stayed the same while the prevalence of obesity has just about doubled compared to 30 years ago (Finucane et al. 2011).

> "Glutton: one who digs his grave with his teeth." (French proverb).

A too-high energy intake leading to weight gain may sometimes be unintentional. In these rather rare cases, the **human intestinal flora** is responsible for this. Depending on their composition, the approximately 50–100 trillion microorganisms living there in symbiosis with our body are capable of recovering energy media – more or less effectively – from the indigestible waste products of our metabolism, e. g. glucose from cellulose. This happens frequently when there is an imbalance in the proportions of bacteria colonizing the intestine, with more inhabitants from the phylum **Firmicutes** and a decreased number from the phylum **Bacteroides**. Dietary modifications can change the intestinal flora rapidly, even within as little as 24 hours (David et al. 2014).

☐ **Fig. 37.1** Source: dpa/akg

38 Fat distribution patterns, their measurands and the risk of dementia

The standard measure of body fat is the body mass index (BMI). It is calculated from the body mass (weight in kg) divided by height in meters squared (m^2). A normal BMI is found in 65 % of 25- to 34-year-old women and in 50 % of the same-aged men. Thirty years later, only approximately one in every three women or men will have a normal weight (◘ Tab. 38.1).

BMI is not the only measurand used to characterize the multiplying number of fat pads in the body. The distribution of the excess adipose tissue is also of great importance. A simple measure of fat distribution patterns is the ratio of waist to hip size. Accordingly, it is harmful to health when this ratio is greater than 0.85 in women and 1.00 in men. An even faster way to determine abdominal obesity is by just measuring the waist circumference alone. The risk of disease increases with a girth of more than 80 cm in women and 94 cm in men and is significantly elevated in circumferences of exceeding 88 and 102 cm, respectively.

An accumulation of fat pads in the abdominal organs, especially in the liver, can also lead to increased mortality rates (▶ Chapter 43). A special measure for estimating the obesity-related mortality hazard is called the ABSI ("a body shape index"). It is calculated from weight, body height and waist circumference (Krakauer et Krakauer 2014).

According to the results of studies conducted in the United States with observation periods spanning several decades, one of the many hazard potentials linked to central obesity (▶ Chapter 39) is the increased risk of dementia (Whitmer et al. 2008, Gelber et al. 2012). Especially obesity in midlife increases this risk (Xu et al. 2011). According to secondary analyses of the Framingham Heart Study, the brain volume of selected patients was lower the higher their BMI (Debette et al. 2010).

In approximately one fifth of overweight and obese persons, the genetically based growth in the number and size of fat cells is evenly distributed and the cells are distributed broadly throughout the subcutaneous compartment (Heid et al. 2010). Because fewer of the visceral biomarkers are released, weight-related health impairments become less manifest in this group of persons.

◘ **Tab. 38.1** Body weight classification in stages according to WHO guidelines

Classification		Body Mass Index (BMI)
Underweight		<18
Normal weight		18.5–24.9
Overweight		25–29.9
Obese	– Class I	30–34.9
	– Class II	35-40.0
	– Class III	>40

39 The site of hormone and messenger substance synthesis: fatty tissue

Obesity causes the growth of fat cells. The release of fatty acids and a variety of diverse cell types that specifically occur in this proportion of fat is facilitated when they come from the especially problematic abdominal adipose tissue. These in turn form dozens of hormones, cytokines and other messenger substances with wide-reaching systemic consequences. Some important bioactive compounds formed in adipose tissue include, among others:

- Adiponectin
- Angiotensin I and II
- Cholesteryl ester transfer protein
- Fetuin-A
- Insulin-like growth factor 1
- Interleukin 1, 6 and 8
- Leptin
- Estradiol
- Plasminogen activator inhibitor-1
- Prostacyclin
- Resistin
- Retinol binding protein 4
- Nitrogen monoxide
- Tumor necrosis factor α
- Vaspin
- Visfatin

The increased production of angiotensin in adipose tissue, for example, is one of the reasons why around 50 % of overweight individuals suffer from too-high blood pressure. Moreover, due to their higher estradiol levels, overweight women are more likely to contract breast and uterine cancer than normal weight women (► Chapter 66), but are less at risk of osteoporosis (► Chapter 76). High leptin levels can lead to degeneration of the joint matrix and subsequently to joint damage (► Chapter 56). The most important obesity-related health-related risks repeatedly confirmed by numerous large international studies (Renehan et al. 2008, Strate et al. 2009, World Cancer Research Fund 2009, Yuan et al. 2013, Sorensen et al. 2014, Wada et al. 2014) are:

- Degenerative joint diseases
- Diabetes mellitus
- Diverticulitis
- Elevated surgical risks
- Bile and kidney stone formation
- Gout
- Myocardial infarction
- Renal damage
- Sleep apnea syndrome
- Stroke
- Phlebitis
- Left atrial enlargement
- Hypertrophy of the left ventricular muscle
- Leukemia
- Multiple myeloma
- Non-Hodgkin lymphoma
- Tumors of the thyroid, esophagus, biliary tract, liver, kidneys, ovaries, prostate and bowel

40 How obesity causes type 2 diabetes

Worldwide, the number of adults with type 2 diabetes has more than doubled since 1980 (Danaei et al. 2011). Why obesity is the main cause for this can be plausibly explained by knowledge of the underlying molecular mechanisms. For example, the **tumor necrosis factor** α produced in the excess fat deposits, the peptide hormone **resistin** as well as the **fetuin-A** given off by fatty livers create an insulin resistance in the muscle cells by blocking the insulin receptors on the cell surfaces. This insulin resistance, together with the associated reduced production of insulin by the β-cells in the pancreas that then usually takes place after a longer period, is what causes type 2 diabetes.

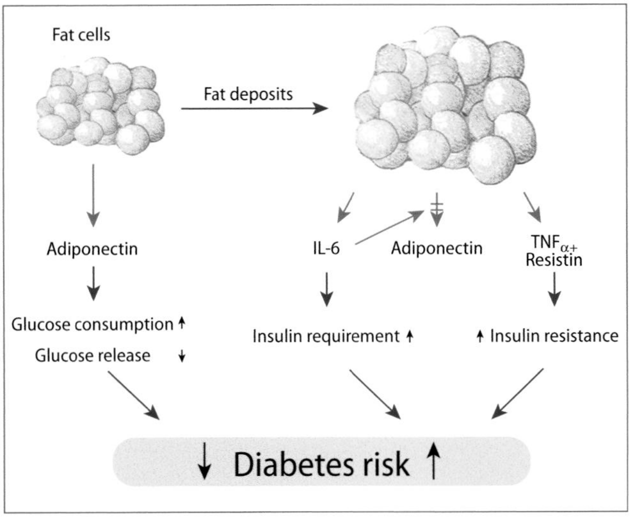

> Type 2 diabetes is the pacing car for cardio-vascular diseases and cancer.

Interleukin 6, also produced by the adipose tissue in chronic inflammation and obesity, is a further risk factor because it stimulates glucose formation in the liver and thereby initiates additional insulin consumption. By contrast, **adiponectin** has previously been thought to be a protection factor, because higher levels of adiponectin are often found when any type 2 diabetes pathology is absent (Li et al. 2009). This initially appears to make sense given that adiponectin stimulates the insulin-independent glucose uptake in the muscle cells and inhibits glucose release in the liver. In actuality, no causal connection exists here. Targeted rises in the adiponectin level do not lower the risk of developing type 2 diabetes (Yaghootkar et al. 2013).

As little as a 10-percent weight reduction markedly improves insulin-sensitivity because the disruption in the normal manifestation of the insulin receptors on the muscle cells can be reversed quickly through persistent work by the muscle.

□ **Fig. 40.1** Molecular mechanism of the development of type 2 diabetes. TNFα tumor necrosis factor α, IL-6 interleukin 6

41 Glycemic index and glycemic load

The **glycemic index (GI)** ranks carbohydrates in food according to the extent to which they raise blood glucose levels after eating. The GI gives a rough estimation as to how quickly a 50-gram serving of a particular food converts to sugar and raises the blood glucose level above normal.

> The steeper the blood glucose level (= glycemia) rises after nutritional intake, the higher the glycemic index.

Foods with a GI lower than 55 lead only to a slight increase in blood glucose levels. As reference, glucose is stated at 100 %. GI values should only be considered a general guideline: GI determinations are subject to large interindividual variability among test subjects, differences in food quality and variations in the way the food is prepared.

The glycemic index was developed by D. Jenkins at the University of Toronto at the beginning of the 1980s to achieve better control for people with diabetes. Furthermore, a high GI gives an indication as to which food will make insulin secretion shoot up, whereby carbohydrates are metabolized into fat faster. In that regard, the glycemic index is similarly helpful for people who want to maintain a healthy diet. But it doesn't say anything about the value of the carbohydrates eaten. Those supplied by fruit, for example, are good because they transport vitamins, secondary plant compounds and dietary fiber. The carbohydrates in table sugar, however, only supply empty calories and can be refrained from.

The GI does not measure the absolute proportion of carbohydrates in a food either. For instance, 50 g of readily digestible energy suppliers are contained in 100 g of white bread, whereas you need 1600 g of carrots to achieve the equivalent. That is why, in many cases, it makes sense to calculate the **glycemic load (GL)** of individual foods (◻ Tab. 41.1). GL, namely, accounts for both the GI and the actual proportion of carbohydrates in 100 g of food. The glycemic load of a defined serving of food is a good way to estimate the body's insulin response directly after the serving is consumed.

> The glycemic load (GL) of a meal is calculated as follows:
> GL = GI × [net carbohydrates (%)/100] × [consumed portion (g)/100]

◘ Tab. 41.1 Glycemic index (GI) and glycemic load (GL) of a few chosen foods

	GI	CHO[a]	GL[b]		GI	CHO[a]	GL[b]
French bread (baguette)	95	50	48	Whole-grain bread	58	46	27
Mashed potatoes	85	13	11	Bananas	52	20	10
Cornflakes	81	87	70	Orange juice	50	11	5.5
French fries	75	20	15	Pumpernickel	50	40	20
Wheat rolls	73	53	39	Cereals	49	66	23
Carrots	70	3	2.1	Macaroni	47	27	13
Couscous	65	23	15	Peaches	42	13	5.5
Brown rice	64	24	15	Ribbon noodles	40	26	10
Raisins	64	72	46	Strawberries	40	3	1.2
Spaghetti	61	25	15	Apples	38	13	4.9
Pineapple	59	11	6.5	Pears	38	9	3.4
Crackers	59	60	35	Beans, white	38	21	8.0
Grapes	59	15	8.9	Yoghurt, natural	36	5	1.8
Soft and fizzy drinks	58	10	5.8	Lentils	29	12	3.5

[a] Carbohydrates in 100 g of food.
[b] Per 100 g portion.

42 Obesity and the risk for disease

In today's society with its nearly unlimited nutritional resources, the survival benefit achieved through the body's ability to store large fat reserves has been reversed (van Cleave et al. 2010). Overweight and obesity are contributing causes to very serious health problems. These include, among others, senile dementia (► Chapter 38), cancer, hypertension, diabetes mellitus and an elevated incidence of arteriosclerotic complications such as myocardial infarction and stroke (Chen et al. 2013, Lu et al. 2014). As demonstrated by the data from a study on 302,296 persons in Europe and the USA with observation periods of 6–35 years, the associated risk, especially for coronary heart disease, increases by 17% in persons with a BMI between 25 and 29.9 and by 45% with a BMI > 30. These figures have already been corrected for the risks of high blood pressure and cholesterol levels (Bogers et al. 2007).

The concurrent presence of cardiovascular diseases and diabetes approximately doubles the risk of death. This association was revealed by the interpretation of a **meta-analysis** (data from comparable studies are amalgamated to strengthen the conclusiveness of their findings) from 102 prospective studies with close to 700,000 patients (ERFC 2010).

The findings of the Nurses' Health Study reinforce the importance of maintaining a normal body weight, starting early in adulthood. In women, extreme obesity at the age of 50 years dramatically limits the perspective for a good state of health at an older age of 70 years (Sun et al. 2009). If obesity

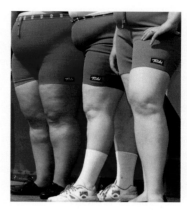

◻ **Fig. 42.1** Source: dpa/akg

sets in at the early age of 18, the chances of staying healthy and strong in older age decrease even further. Each kilogram of weight gain after the 18th year of life decreases these chances by 5%.

One particular characteristic is repeatedly described by larger studies. In patients who are already severely ill, e.g. suffer from chronic kidney disease, diabetes, cardiovascular disease or cancer, the ones with a higher BMI will often have better survival chances than leaner patients (Carnethon et al. 2012, Sharma et al. 2014). This phenomenon is termed **the obesity paradox** in the literature. Many theories have been suggested to explain the underlying physiology, but it still remains unclear (Angeras et al. 2013, von Haehling et al. 2013, de Schutter et al. 2014).

43 Obesity and mortality risk

According to the data from many large-scale studies, marked obesity is associated with an increased risk of mortality (Greenberg 2013). A meta-analysis of prospective studies on this subject gave special consideration to the age, sex and smoking status of 894,576 participants (Whitlock et al. 2009). The findings showed that obesity, reflected in a BMI between 30 and 35, reduced life expectancy by 2–4 years. A total of 8–10 years of life were lost when the person's weight produced a BMI between 40 and 45. The latter decreased life expectancy is approximately equal to the effect of smoking. Another large meta-analysis by the National Cancer Institutes in the USA covering 19 prospective studies with data from nearly 1.5 million adults of European origin and observation periods of 5–28 years yielded the same results (Gonzales et al. 2010).

Since BMI is not the most optimal measure for determining the amount of abdominal fat mass that can cause illness, overweight persons with fat mass distributed over the whole body or very muscular athletes even with a BMI of 25–29.9 can have a longer life expectancy than people with normal weight (Flegal et al. 2013). Conversely, when the accumulation of fat pads in the abdominal organs and especially in the liver becomes too large, the mortality rates are higher, even in normal-weight or underweight persons (Zhang et al. 2008, Cerhan et al. 2014). The results of the Framingham Heart Study (Britton et al. 2013) and the EPIC study (van der A et al. 2014) have confirmed that large amounts of abdominal fat are related to higher mortality rates.

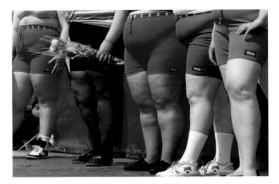

◘ **Fig. 43.1** Source: dpa/akg

A too high proportion of abdominal fat minimized by surgical interventions can confer significant health benefits (Adams et al. 2012, O'Brien et al. 2013). This was also shown by the Swedish Obese Subjects Study, ongoing since 1981, concerning the relationship between body weight and mortality (Sjöström et al. 2007, 2012, 2014, Carlsson et al. 2012). The authors used interventions based on bariatric surgery to lower the weight of people with morbid obesity. In these patients, they performed gastric bypass surgery, which leaves only a smaller portion of the stomach remaining for nutritional uptake, or they shortened their intestine. Then, they compared this study population with a cohort of obese controls who did not undergo surgery. Only those patients who underwent surgery achieved substantial weight loss and had a markedly reduced incidence of type 2 diabetes, myocardial infarction and stroke, as well as lower overall mortality.

44 Intentional weight loss

Weight reduction should be slow and steady because our body is not aware of our intended diet. It reacts to the food scarcity as it would react to starvation, immediately lowering the energy requirement for the organ basic functions (▶ Chapter 8). Fast weight losses are generally only transient and almost always lead to weight fluctuations that are harmful to health. According to the results produced to date by an EU-funded study in 8 countries, such yo-yo effects can be best minimized by diets with a moderately high protein content and modestly reduced glycemic index (Larsen et al. 2010).

A simple and frequently successful recommendation for committed dieters is to sensibly enjoy their food by being more conscious of what they're eating. That said, it takes approx. 30 minutes, namely, before the hormonal feedback circuitry sends the satiety signal from the stomach and intestine to the center in the hypothalamus (▶ Chapter 13). To avoid disappointment, an achievable weight loss goal of 5 kg per 150 days should be set. The ratio of body surface area to body mass over which energy is expended as heat is smaller in obese people. That is why they tend to lose weight more slowly than their lean counterparts. However, even small weight loss brings health benefits because the risk-associated abdominal fat is always broken down first and at a disproportionately faster rate.

Indeed, a low-fat meal is just as satisfying as the same amount of fat-rich fare. Such deliberations are important, seeing as when as little as only 5 g of the recommended carbohydrate uptake is replaced with 5 g of fat it leads to a weight gain of a good kilogram every year even though the amount of food eaten remains the same. Therefore, every person with weight problems is recommended to reduce their daily fat intake (Hooper et al. 2012). Fundamentally, this nutrient proportion should make up no more than 30% of the total caloric intake and should consist of 1/3 saturated, 1/3 monounsaturated and 1/3 polyunsaturated fatty acids (▶ Chapter 5 and ▶ Chapter 15).

> Dieting based on rigid behavioral controls or strict bans is not very helpful. Rather, it tends to lead to further eating disorders.

One concept of the presently heated debate on restricting calories and occasional fasting is that of **autophagy**. In this natural form of "self-digestion", the body's cells breakdown damaged or no longer required components to produce new energy equivalents or other molecules required for cellular metabolism. Thus, autophagy is not only an emergency system that kicks in during starvation phases. It is also responsible for the constant cleaning and renewal of cells (Oh et Lee 2012, Rubinsztein et al. 2012). Bacteria and viruses are similarly subject to this "spring cleaning" process. Therefore, autophagy is also a central player in our immune system (Bhattacharya et Eissa 2013). This cleaning process ensures maintenance of healthy cells and cell functions. Good recycling can therefore prolong life, but only functions on low nutritional input. That said, when we eat the 5–6 snacks and main meals we do every day, insulin is secreted constantly. However, insulin inhibits autophagy. Occasional fasting and a maximum of 2–3 meals per day in conjunction with physical activity (▶ Chapter 59), however, promote the desired effect of cellular neogenesis owing to the comparatively low insulin levels.

45 Special features of diets

Statistically, people in the industrialized countries consume between 130–150 g fat every day, whereas only around 90–110 g is justifiable from a long-term health perspective, depending on the individual's caloric needs. However, for many, it is often difficult sticking to within these limits. Indeed, many foodstuffs or cafeteria food frequently contain fat content that is not listed on the label. And a load of fat is hidden where you would least expect it, i. e. as much as up to 8 % in whole grain bread. But not only do we eat too much fat, we mostly eat animal fat, i. e. the wrong kind of fat that contains saturated fatty acids.

10 g fat (saturated fatty acids) are contained in:
- 2/3 croissant
- 2 yogurt bars (25 g)
- 16 potato chips
- 20 g roasted peanuts
- 20 g chocolate
- 32 g whipping cream
- 4 cups of mélange coffee

Too high fat intake can cause overweight. Unfortunately, the diets that invariably follow are usually associated with problems of malnutrition.

In this context, for instance, diets are constantly propagated that allow unlimited fat consumption, but reduce consumption of carbohydrates in compensation. From the perspective of losing weight, this might appear to constitute a rather promising strategy at first glance. This ties in with the fact that most people tend to dislike eating large amounts of fat without consuming them simultaneously with carbohydrates, thereby also very reliably lowering their energy uptake. This leads to quick initial success, which is how the likes of the Atkins diet earned their popularity. All large studies on this topic have shown, however, that weight loss from a diet lasting a year and longer is solely dictated by the duration and the restriction of calories and not from the choice of energy transfer media.

Irrespective of the above, fat-rich diets are always harmful due to the unbridled uptake of saturated fatty acids and the associated elevation in cholesterol biosynthesis.

Effective weight reduction programs always go hand-in-hand with a sensible change in nutrition-related habits. This includes a balanced diet consisting of abundant complex carbohydrates e.g. in fruits, vegetables, potatoes and grains. These are carriers of minerals, trace elements, bioactive plant compounds, dietary fiber and most vitamins. In this context, note should be taken of the fact that, unlike complex carbohydrates, simple carbohydrates in the form of sugar are mere energy suppliers. The daily intake of sugar, e.g. from honey, jam, sweet baked goods, sweet drinks, chocolate, other sweets or hidden in various convenience meals and/or food additives, should therefore be limited to a maximum of 10 % (approx. 50–75 g sugar) of the respective recommended daily energy intake (WHO 2009).

46 Nutrigenomics

Everybody adapts differently to its nutritional opportunities. This will make the future of nutrition very exciting once the field of **nutrigenomics**, a still young branch of medicine, has fully established itself. The aim of this multidisciplinary science is to find out how nutrients in the foods we eat affect gene regulation. It appears that, owing to evolution, nutrients interfere in genetic activities and thereby in interlinked protein biosynthesis processes. Such alterations in protein synthesis occurring in an individual, in turn, affect metabolism in their liver, gut and muscles, and may perhaps cause illnesses or, conversely, promote robust health (Sales et al. 2014).

One well-known example of genetically induced intolerability of a food is lactose intolerance. Over the millennia of dairy cattle breeding, a genetic variant has prevailed in nearly 90 % of the people in Europe that helps them continue to be able to digest lactose into adulthood without any problems. This confers a great survival benefit because milk and milk products are considered very healthy – when tolerated. In a small proportion of Europeans and in most Africans and Asians, however, the gene for lactose breakdown is switched off in early childhood. That is why the intake of milk products makes them sick.

Glucosinolates are another interesting example for how our diet is driven by our genes, at least in part (▶ Chapter 25). In some people, these secondary plant compounds, like those occurring in cress, radish or mustard among others, strongly inhibit the formation of thyroid hormones. Some afflicted persons, however, have an unusual mutation in the taste receptors on their tongues that causes them

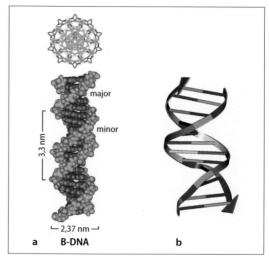

■ **Fig. 46.1** Model-like representation of the basic structure of genes

to taste vegetables containing glucosinolates as extremely bitter. Therefore, these people avoid such types of vegetables, thereby protecting themselves from their harmful side effects.

In other words, our genes often determine what tastes good to us and what is well-tolerated. Therefore, every individual should find out for themselves which foods are good for them in terms of health-related aspects. If the future brings us a better understanding of the functional interactions between diet and genes, the use of optimized foodstuffs and personalized nutritional regimens will help us markedly lower the risk for many chronic diseases.

II Exercise

47 No sports?

The WHO estimates that, by the year 2020, our lifestyle will be a co-factor responsible for around 70 % of all diseases. One major problem is the lack of exercise stemming from the changes in our world, i.e. sitting too long every day at the workplace and during our leisure time (▶ Chapter 85). Indeed, the skeletal muscles are not only involved in exercise. they are also an important metabolic organ. During physical activities, a variety of immunological and hormonal messenger substances are produced in the working muscles which then affect the central circuitry of our bodies. These substances, called myokines, have a very positive influence on the duration and quality of our lives (Kvaavik et al. 2010, Pedersen et Febbraio 2012, Bente 2013).

> Exercise is extremely important for all bodily functions.

The effects conferred by physical activity on improving health and extending survival can be observed well into old age (Hamer et al. 2014). According to the results of an older prospective long-term study with approx. 17,000 person-years, most of the 70-, 78- and 85 year-old test subjects who engaged in at least 4 hours of physical activity per week lived markedly longer than their lazier peers (Stessman et al. 2009).

Physical activity might even slow down the aging process of the genes. This evidence was provided by a study that investigated **telomere length** in 2,401 twins aged 18–81 (Cherkas et al. 2008).

Telomeres consist of tandemly repeated DNA sequences at the end of the chromosomes that do not give any building instructions to the body. However, they protect the gene strands from committing errors during duplication. Telomere length, especially in the white blood corpuscles, and the magnitude of their natural shortening with every cell division are indicators for biological aging in humans. In the test subjects of the same calendar age who engaged in a good 3 hours of physical activity per week, the telomeres averaged 200 nucleotides longer than in their unathletic twins. Because the telomere length in leukocytes declines by an average of 21 nucleotides per year, these 200 nucleotides prove that the physically active individuals were biologically approximately 10 years younger than their inactive peers. Apparently, telomere length is a general measure of health. One result of the Nurses' Health Study showed that women with a healthy lifestyle had longer leukocyte telomeres than women with an unhealthy lifestyle (Sun et al. 2012). The health benefits of longer telomeres that have actually been measurable to date include findings that the risk of both cancer incidence and mortality is statistically significantly lowered (Willeit et al. 2010).

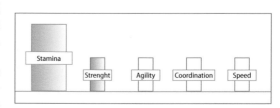

◼ **Fig. 47.1** Training objectives in sports

48 The outstanding merits of endurance

Aerobic dynamic endurance exercise causing the working muscles to contract and relax continuously and repeatedly is nearly always the basis for athletic success: regardless of whether it's top athletes competing for medals or recreational athletes pursing enjoyment and promoting their fitness level. Nowadays, remarkable endurance undertakings are very popular: running, hiking, walking, cycling, rowing, swimming, inline skating, mountain climbing, skiing and dancing.

Lifestyle, health status, social environment and local circumstances are factors key to selecting the type of exercise to engage in. The many options for exercise give everyone the chance to derive pleasure from engaging in physical activity.

However, the more sedentary among us tend to lack the willpower to engage in physical activity. We have gotten out of touch with our own bodies. Frequently, we demand too much of them at the same time. Our musculoskeletal system alerts us to pain, we sustain injuries. rapidly our interest wanes. Anyone wanting to pursue such a radical life-changing process is therefore recommended to start with moderate physical exercise. It is necessary to take each individual's own methods, age, gender, experience, talent, weight, psyche and general state of health into consideration. The most important aspect is **to exercise regularly**.

The pulse rates recommended by the European Atherosclerosis Society for the "sports weaned" can be taken as a general guideline for suitable exertion limits:

- 20–29 years: 115–145
- 30–39 years: 110–140
- 40–49 years: 105–130
- 50–59 years: 100–125
- 60–69 years: 95–115

Once a good level of physical fitness has been attained, the frequency and then the extent of the endurance exercises should be increased further. For health maintenance, the WHO recommends that adults engage in 150 minutes of endurance sports a week, distributed over 3–5 days (WHO 2014). According to data from a large prospective study on 3.45 million person-years of follow-up, just 15 minutes of moderate-intensity exercise a day can confer life expectancy benefits (Wen et al. 2011).

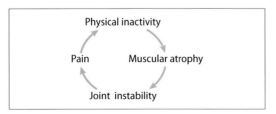

◘ Fig. 48.1 Consequences of physical inactivity

The "often, longer, intensive" rule: First train more often, then also longer and then increase the intensity. Simultaneous increases in scope and intensity of training only make sense in athletes with very high levels of physical fitness.

49 Endurance sports and the heart

Physical activity has important positive effects on the heart. Depending on its exercise-related output, the myocardium can grow from 300 g up to 500 g, the chamber volume expand from 600 ml up to 1300 ml. The chamber walls thicken by up to 20 % and the heart beat volume rises from 60 up to 110 ml. In aggregate, this economization of cardiac output leads to a reduction in blood pressure and heart rate.

According to reports published by the European Society of Cardiology, the following 5 risk factors cause three-quarters of all severe **heart diseases:**

- Smoking
- Diabetes
- Hypertension
- High LDL cholesterol
- Low HDL cholesterol

The Society therefore recommended in 2012:

- Avoid consuming tobacco in any form whatsoever
- Eat a varied diet, with low-saturated fats, but with many whole-grain products, vegetables, fruit and fish
- 2.5–5 hours of moderate intensive physical activity per week
- Blood pressure levels under 140/90 mmHg
- Lowering too-high LDL cholesterol levels (▶ Chapter 18)

The importance of these recommendations is reflected in the confirmatory findings of the Whitehall II study ongoing since 1985 (Hardoon et al. 2011).

In relation to cardiovascular diseases, people benefit immensely from the risk-reducing effect of physical activity – women and men in equal measure (Hamer et al. 2014). In one United States study on 11,049 men over an average observation period of 25 years, cardiovascular disease mortality in elderly men with high fitness levels was approximately halved compared to those test subjects with low fitness levels (Berry et al. 2011). In patients with coronary heart disease or in rehabilitation after a stroke, physical activity is just as good as or even better than medicines (Naci et Ioannidis 2013).

The resting pulse of people who do not get any exercise is usually too fast (▶ Chapter 50). Among others, this increases the risk of myocardial infarction, as shown by the analyses of the Women's Health Initiative on 129,135 participating menopausal women (Hsia et al. 2009). The connection between heart rate and mortality exists in younger people and similarly applies to men. One large Norwegian study investigated this aspect, monitoring 50,088 persons aged from 20 years for over 18 years. A resting heart rate of 101 beats per minute increases the risk of death in men by 73 % compared to men with a resting heart rate of 61–72 beats (Nauman et al. 2010).

50 Endurance training and heart rate

The resting heart rate is defined as the heart rate measured immediately after a night's rest, while still lying down. In adults, it is approximately 70 beats per minute. Endurance training lowers the heart rate to around 60 beats per minute in most recreational sports enthusiasts, 50 beats per minute in amateur athletes and often as low as 35–40 beats per minute in high-performance athletes. High body temperature (fever) increases the heart rate. a one degree increase in body temperature causes ten extra heartbeats. Measuring your resting heart rate is therefore a useful tool to check on your general health status. If your resting pulse is raised by more than 8 beats per minute in the morning, your exercise routine should be reduced or completely stopped.

> The optimal heart rate during endurance exercise is between 60 and 85 % of the maximum achievable heart rate.

In healthy persons, the maximum heart rate achieved during physical activity is age-dependent (Larson et al. 2013). It is approximately calculated by 220 minus age. Any personal training program should be based on this calculation.

This equates to walking at a fast pace while still being able to talk without difficulty. The correlation between heart rate and degree of physical activity is nearly linear at a heart rate range of around 120–170, which is useful when devising training programs.

It is sometimes useful to check your heart rate during physical activity. Ideally, this should be measured using small devices attached to the body. Heart rate measurements checked manually have the disadvantage that physical activity must be interrupted, limiting accuracy. It takes several seconds to accurately check your pulse when resting, during which time it will have already slowed down.

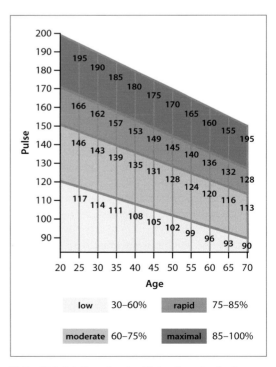

◻ **Fig. 50.1** Relation of workout intensity and pulse for different age groups

51 Endurance training and the large blood vessels

Regular exercise increases the blood volume in the veins and arteries, which in turn improves the viscosity of the blood because it lowers the concentrations of clotting factors like fibrinogens while increasing the amount of tissue-specific plasminogen activators. The transportation of oxygen and temperature regulation are improved.

The interior surface of the blood vessels, the **endothelium**, also plays a key role in improving blood vessel function during regular endurance exercise. This cell layer then produces more **nitrogen monoxide** and **prostacyclin** (▶ Chapter 15). Both substances cause the blood vessels to dilate and, as a result, lower the blood pressure. Furthermore, prostacyclin inhibits platelet activation, thereby also reducing the risk of thrombosis. Finally, fewer inflammatory cells migrate into the blood vessel wall, which in turn is linked to a reduction in the arteriosclerosis risk.

The increased blood flow during exercise is thought to cause an increase in endothelial activity (Flammer et al. 2012). Its intensity can be easily measured by ultrasound as flow-mediated vasodilation, or FMD for short, and is a parameter for assessing endothelial function. The higher the elasticity of the arteries, the better the condition of the endothelium and the lower the risk of coronary heart disease and hypertension becomes (▶ Chapter 53).

In general, too much abdominal fat can reduce the FMD of the arteries (Romero-Corral et al. 2010).

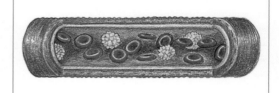

◻ Fig. 51.1

Endurance athletes therefore also benefit from their strenuous exercise in terms of optimal endothelial function because they usually do not suffer from excessive accumulations of body fat. With minor limitations, these dual benefits of endurance training similarly apply to overweight people: When they engage in physical exercise their visceral fat deposits tend to be burned off first (▶ Chapter 56). The Women's Health Study conducted on 10,339 women over a mean observation period of 14 years showed that regular physical activity could considerably reduce the risk for hypertension in overweight women. However, these findings could not be transferred completely to the risk profile of normal-weight women (Jackson et al. 2014).

The large blood vessels also benefit from plenty of exercise.

52 Endurance training and the capillaries

The key benefits of physical activity and exercise are:
- Capillary neogenesis
- Opening of resting capillaries
- Formation of collateral circulation
- Maintaining elasticity
- Widening of the lumen

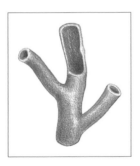

Fig. 52.1

Neogenesis of capillaries occurs specifically in the working muscles. This improves the oxidative capacity given that it increases the volume of the mitochondria at the same time. **Mitochondria** are the cells' power houses where energy is generated via the citrate cycle and the respiratory chain (▶ Chapter 6). The cell's metabolism becomes more effective in that less oxygen is consumed to achieve the same output.

To wit, the blood pressure elevation during physical activity increases capillary density, dilates resting capillaries and leads to the formation of **a collateral circulation** ("watershed effect"). Blood volume is more effectively distributed and energy is generated by the citric acid cycle and respiratory

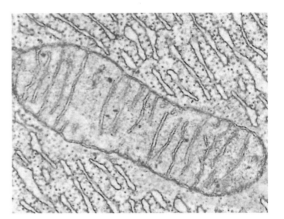

Fig. 52.2 Electron microscopic recording of a mitochondrion

chain (▶ Chapter 6). Cell metabolism becomes more effective by reducing the oxygen demand for the same level of exertion.

The higher blood pressure during physical activity produces an increase in capillary density and resting oxygen supply is better utilized. The vessels remain more elastic. An exercise regimen of more than 5 hours per week widens the blood vessel lumen, significantly increases localized blood flow and markedly lowers the resting blood pressure (▶ also Chapter 53).

53 Endurance training and blood pressure

Blood pressure results from the regulated interplay between the heart and the blood vessels. It fluctuates significantly, with higher readings during physical activity than at rest, and is higher during the day than at night. Blood pressure consists of two phases: the systole, when the heart muscle contracts, and the diastole, when the heart muscle relaxes. Arterial hypertension occurs when the blood pressure in the arterial system is permanently elevated. in lay terms, it is simply called **high blood pressure**. According to the WHO, arterial hypertension is defined as a systolic blood pressure equal to or above 140 mmHg and/or a diastolic pressure equal to or above 90 mmHg. The results of a Swedish study of 1.2 million men, observed over 24 years, suggest that a higher diastolic pressure poses an increased risk in young adults, whereas the systolic blood pressure is more relevant in older individuals (Sundström et al. 2011).

The lack of early warning symptoms is the really confounding part about this disease. High blood pressure often remains undiagnosed for years and causes significant, irreversible damage over time. This includes, among other things, vascular damage with the possible development of coronary heart disease, myocardial infarction, stroke, ocular and renal damage or dementia. Nearly half of all deaths in under-65-year-olds are associated with hypertension-related diseases (◘ Tab. 53.1).

Blood pressure is regulated by hormones via the **renin-angiotensin-aldosterone system**. About 30 % of the adult population in Germany is permanently affected by hypertension, and more than 1 in 5 adults worldwide. Early diagnosis in young adults would be possible and useful, but seldom happens (Allen

◘ **Tab. 53.1** Blood pressure classification (WHO)

	Systolic (mmHg)	Diastolic (mmHg)
Optimal blood pressure	<120	<80
Normal blood pressure	120–129	80–84
High normal blood pressure (Prehypertension)	130–139	85–89
Stage 1 hypertension	140–159	90–99
Stage 2 hypertension	160–179	100–109
Stage 3 hypertension (hypertensive emergency)	>180	>110
Isolated systolic hypertension	>140	<90

et al. 2014). High blood pressure is treated with medication, although it is very important that those afflicted change their lifestyle as well. This includes weight reduction, increasing the consumption of fruit and vegetables, cooking with unsaturated fats, **reducing salt intake,** restricting sugary drinks, giving up smoking, restricting alcohol intake and avoiding long-term stress (Aburto et al. 2013, Mancia et al. 2013, Yokoyama et al. 2014).

Physical exercise is a paramount component of basic therapy. It is mainly endurance training that promote the cardiovascular system. Regular exercise leads to a long-term reduction in systolic values by about 10–15 mmHg and in diastolic values by about 5–10 mmHg (► Chapter 49 to ► Chapter 51). The involvement of a sports physician should be compulsory.

54 Endurance training and the lungs

The key benefits of physical activity and exercise are:

- Reduction in respiratory rate
- Increased gas exchange surface
- Optimized ventilation

A healthy adult at rest breathes between 10 and 14 times per minute. The gas volume per breath, known as tidal volume, is between 500–1000 ml. A rule of thumb for calculating tidal volume is body weight in kg × 10 to 15.

Respiratory rate and **tidal volume** are age- and height-dependent. The product of both is the **total ventilation**. This reflects the total volume of gas exchanged per minute and is about 7–14 liters, but can increase up to 80 during high levels of physical activity and up to 120 liters under extreme exertion. For example, 7 liters of air contain about 1.5 liters of oxygen. The uptake by the lungs is about 300 ml. When consuming a mixed diet (► Chapter 5), the respiratory quotient is 0.89, meaning around 270 ml of carbon dioxide is released.

> The respiratory quotient (RQ) is the ratio of carbon dioxide given off to oxygen volume absorbed. This quotient varies depending on the energy source metabolized because the oxygen demand for the 3 basic nutrients differs. Carbohydrates (RQ = 1), fat (RQ = 0.7), protein (RQ = 0.81).

Two percent of the oxygen absorbed is needed purely for the effort of the respiratory muscles at rest. This can increase ten-fold during high-level physical activity. The benefits of regular endurance training are a lower respiratory rate and an increased gas exchange surface. Breathing is optimized and lung function improved. In patients with asthma, the threshold of an exercise-induced attack is raised.

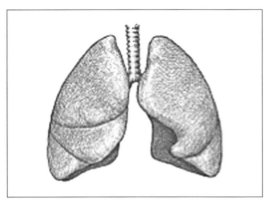

◘ Fig. 54.1

55 Endurance training and the brain

Even during moderate physical activity, cerebral blood circulation is 30 % higher. Rigorous physical activity is the best way to maintain the body's nearly **100 billion** brain cells and improve their function by enabling the brain to develop a variety of new synapses. In an adult, every single nerve cell has on average around 1000 such connections to other nerve cells. The total number of these synapses is around **100 trillion**. As a result of sport, thought processes become easier, and intelligence, learning and memory are optimally enhanced. The hippocampus, the central region of the brain controlling memory and spatial orientation, undergoes less age-induced atrophy when the elderly regularly engage in adequate physical activity (Smith et al. 2014).

The improved **cerebral metabolism** leads to greater production of hundreds of chemicals, including nerve growth factors such as brain-derived neurotropic factor (BDNF), which is deficient in depression. Dopamine, serotonin and noradrenaline are some of the many neurotransmitters produced. Of special interest is the up to four-fold increase in the release of endogenous opioids, called endorphins. These are primarily formed in the frontal lobe of the cerebral cortex and the limbic system. Both areas of the brain play a key role in the **processing of feelings** and in **pain suppression**. Physical activity confers considerable psychological benefits to well-being, higher self-esteem, the release of pent-up aggression, a distancing from exaggerated problems, mitigating negative feelings and a general resistance to stress. Caution is advised in contact sports because repetitive blows to the head can

cause minor damage to the brain (Koerte et al. 2012, McAllister et al. 2014).

> Regular exercise stimulates thought processes.

Obesity, often associated with physical inactivity in middle age, increases the risk of dementia (▶ Chapter 38). Insulin resistance, similar to that in diabetics, plays an important role in this. People with diabetes thus have a 60–90 % higher risk of dementia compared to the normal population. According to the findings of current studies, people who are physically active in their youth and engage in lifelong exercise, and those who follow a diet rich in fish, poultry, nuts, salad, fruit and vegetables with limited intake of fat and cow meat (▶ Chapter 32), cannot only reduce minor age-associated cognitive impairment, but also significantly reduce their risk for dementia (Gu et al. 2010, Middleton et al. 2010, Ahlskog et al. 2011, DeFina et al. 2013).

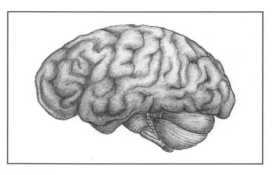

◘ Fig. 55.1

56 Endurance training and fatty tissue

The key benefits of physical activity and exercise are:
- Breaking down excessive fatty tissue with significant benefits on metabolism and the cardiovascular system
- Reducing the incidence of chronic diseases
- General reduction in body weight, which in turn relieves pressure on the joints – all associated with enhanced psychological well-being

Regular exercise lowers triglyceride levels. When fatty tissue is broken down, abdominal fat is reduced first. This has a positive effect given that abdominal fatty tissue is particularly damaging to health (▶ Chapter 38 and ▶ Chapter 39).

Cholesterol levels change very little as a result of physical activity. The findings of numerous randomized, controlled studies show a slight increase in HDL cholesterol levels and a slight decrease in LDL cholesterol levels. The LDL particles increase in size as a result of endurance sport, which helps to reduce the risk of atherosclerosis as small LDL particles carry a higher risk (▶ Chapter 18).

The majority of all hip and knee replacements can be linked to overweight and obesity (Anandacoomarasamy et al. 2009, Wang et al. 2009, Smith et al. 2014).

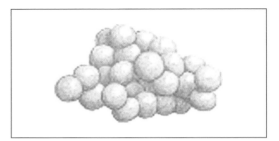

◘ Fig. 56.1

The aesthetic effect should not be underestimated either. The reduction in waistline resulting from more exercise considerably reinforces people's general self-esteem.

It is not just the excess weight that is responsible for the joint damage but also the hormone leptin produced by the fatty tissue (▶ Chapter 13). This can damage the joint cartilage by causing chronic low-grade inflammation. The breakdown of fatty tissue caused by endurance training therefore has *a twofold* benefit for the joints. There is less weight on them and less leptin to damage them.

57 Endurance training and hormones

Metabolism's natural role is the provision of energy equivalents in the form of ATP molecules (► Chapter 6) and in the synthesis of building blocks for the many biochemical cellular processes. The complex network of reactions needed for this is regulated by different control mechanisms. Hormones are important elements in these coordination processes. They act as endogenous messengers that are released into the blood stream and achieve important biological effects within minutes or hours. The hormones are produced on demand in the endocrine glands or in specialized tissue. They only have an effect on certain organs or tissue. Only these particular target organs have receptors that bind hormones, which then become active. Unimaginably small amounts, often less than a hundred-thousandth of a gram per liter, are required.

The main hormones regulating energy production (metabolism) are **glucagon, growth hormone, glucocorticoids,** the **thyroid hormones** as well as **adrenaline** and **insulin.** These enable the body to perform strenuous physical activity by keeping glucose levels in the blood at a normal level. Falling levels of these hormones are a signal for fatigue. Regular training triggers important adaptation processes associated with their secretion.

In this context, glucagon is the antagonist of insulin. It is produced in the pancreas and mobilizes the body's energy reserves, for example, by increasing the neogenesis of glucose from amino acids in the liver. Its secretion is triggered when the blood glucose level falls to under 50 mg/100 ml.

As its name suggests, growth hormone increases muscle growth and reduces the amino acid concentration in the blood by increasing protein synthesis. Furthermore, it enables the body to adjust its metabolism more easily during states of hunger by reducing the peripheral use of glucose and increasing the availability of fatty acids as an energy source via lipolysis of fatty tissue.

Other important hormones in this context are the glucocorticoids (steroid hormones) produced in the adrenal cortex.

> Glucocorticoids protect the body from the negative effects of on-going stresses. These include hunger, thirst, extreme temperature, injury, infection and severe physical or psychological stress.

Cortisol is the most important of these hormones. It slows down glucose metabolism in the peripheral tissue and activates glucose synthesis in the liver. As amino acids are required, it also leads to protein degradation particularly in muscles and bones. Sometimes the lymphatic tissue can also be affected by the breakdown of proteins. This can lead to reduced antibody production with negative consequences for the immune system.

Similarly, the thyroid hormones have a considerable effect on metabolism. They drive protein synthesis, glucose re-absorption in the gut, glucose release from glycogen in the liver and muscles and mobilize fatty acids from fat deposits. The actions of adrenaline and insulin are discussed in ► Chapter 58 and ► Chapter 59.

58 Energy metabolism and the action of adrenaline

At the start of physical exercise, signals from the central nervous system (brain), in particular the hypothalamus, as well as from the muscles used, activate the hormone system. This means that the pituitary gland releases **ACTH** (adrenocorticotropic hormone), **STH** (growth hormone) and **ADH** (antidiuretic hormone) or the adrenal medulla releases the catecholamines **adrenaline** and **noradrenaline** by activating the sympathetic nervous system.

These signal hormones either have a direct effect or regulate the release of secondary hormones via a feedback loop. The intensity of the hormonal response to physical stimuli varies in individuals, and depends on their health status, diet, the menstrual cycle phase in women and, not least, on general fitness. During shorter training periods at a constant level, hormonal reactions are usually diminished. By contrast, endurance training can intensify the activity of some hormones.

Adrenaline is one example of this intensified effect. It is released in larger amounts in highly fit athletes during peak physical exertion. Adrenaline suppresses insulin secretion and enhances glucagon synthesis while keeping the blood sugar level sufficiently high during periods of exertion. Depending on the intensity of physical activity, the fat burned in the muscle increases because of the lipolytic effect of adrenaline, which is supported by glucagon and glucocorticoids, making high plasma levels of fatty acids available.

The benefit of adrenaline on energy metabolism is further enhanced by its central stimulating effect and its ability to improve the contractility of the heart and skeletal muscles. The latter, in particular, affects actual athletic performance as well as conferring long-term benefits. Adrenaline levels at rest reduce with increasing age. Therefore, endurance training stimulates repeatedly higher secretion of adrenaline, providing relative protection for the muscles from early ageing.

59 Energy metabolism and the action of insulin

While adrenaline release varies in an exercise-dependent way, **insulin levels** initially remain normal during exercise, but decrease during longer periods of activity. As glucose utilization is considerably increased during physical activity, trained athletes need less insulin for a particular amount of glucose. One reason for this is that regular physical activity improves the effectiveness of insulin binding to the insulin receptors in the muscle cells. Another reason is that **hormone-independent transporter mechanisms** used for glucose uptake in the cells are boosted during exercise.

> Muscular contractions in and of themselves can stimulate access to intramuscular glucose reserves.

Under these conditions, the only process that insulin still fully controls is that of mobilizing extramuscular glucose depots for use by the muscles (see ▶ Chapter 58).

The fact that insulin release is lower during physical activity may initially come as a surprise. Upon closer scrutiny, however, it becomes clear that this is another useful adaptation mechanism nature has equipped the human body with – namely to its energy metabolism. Consider the following theoretical scenario: high insulin secretion during physical activity would prevent the necessary endogenous glucose synthesis from being initiated in the liver and the exercise session would have to be cut short. If, on top of that, there were an exercise-stimulus-triggered, insulin-independent influx of glucose into the muscle cell, this would result in an ongoing risk of hypoglycemia with serious impairments to health.

> Lower insulin levels during physical exertion promote cellular cleansing and rejuvenation (Chapter 44).

60 Energy optimization for high performance requirements

Glycogen stores, immensely important in endurance training, normally last for up to 1.5 hours. When physical demands become greater, a change in daily eating habits is required. That would mean adding slightly more carbohydrates (up to 60–65 % of the diet) as needed to keep the glycogen reserves at a constant level. Taking this to the next level, athletes aiming to prepare for a specific challenge, for example, to run a marathon, can try to increase their carbohydrate reserves in the liver and muscles by following a special diet. This can be achieved quite effectively by reducing the protein and fat intake over a few days. Then, 4 days before the sporting event, either by completing an exhausting activity or by including a day of fasting, followed by 3 days consuming a diet of mainly carbohydrates such as pasta, rice, grains, fruit and vegetables that are easy to digest.

> This carbohydrate loading can increase the normal reserves in the liver and muscle from 80 to 350g.

However, this kind of carbohydrate loading is not suitable for everyone. A large amount of carbohydrates can cause digestive problems including diarrhea. It can also cause a shock when one steps on and tips the scales. Three grams of water are stored per extra gram of carbohydrates. That is why body weight increases by about half a kilogram. It is always advisable to first try out these short-term dietary changes to ensure they are tolerated.

The timing of the last food intake prior to physical activity is, of course, not just a random decision. In general, it is beneficial to fast for 2–3 hours before physical exertion in the morning. Athletes can avoid excessive insulin secretion by taking readily absorbable glucose or sugar 1–2 hours before starting sports. These sugar-induced insulin peaks are not unusual after nocturnal fasting without breakfast the following morning. They often reduce performance because they can cause hypoglycemia and inhibit the burning of fat immediately before exercise.

61 Endurance training and immunity

The key benefits of physical activity and exercise are:
- Activation of natural killer cells, granulocytes, macrophages and acute-phase proteins (= nonspecific immunity)
- Improved phagocytosis of the immune cells
- Development of tolerance to oxidative stress

Natural killer cells are large lymphocytes that primarily attack and destroy virus-infected cells and tumor cells, but also transplanted foreign tissue. As with T lymphocytes, cytotoxic capacity is driven by perforin and granzymes. During illness, a rise in cell count takes place within 24 hours. This rise lasts for 1–3 days and normalizes again after 5–7 days.

Granulocytes mobilize the fastest. They directly breakdown antigens with their peroxidase system. In bacterial infections, the number of granulocytes can increase up to two- to six-fold.

Macrophages, so-called scavenger cells, connect their toll-like receptors to the pathogens, digesting them and thus making them available as antigen-presenting cells to the lymphocytes.

Acute-phase proteins (APP) act as pattern recognition receptors. They connect to the molecular structure of the pathogens so that they are recognized by the granulocytes or macrophages. The C-reactive protein is one of these APPs. Its levels can rise to several times the norm during physical activity, depending on the intensity, but are usually lower than normal in athletes at rest (Swardfager et al. 2012).

The development of a tolerance to oxidative stress is possible because of the increased activity of those enzymes which reduce oxidative stress. Compared to non-athletic persons, lower amounts of reactive oxygen compounds are measured in endurance athletes (▶ Chapter 27).

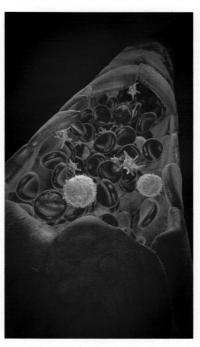

◻ **Fig. 61.1** Capillary vessel with erythrocytes, leukocytes, thrombocytes. (© Dermatzke/fotolia.com)

62 Moderate endurance training and non-specific immunity

During roughly the first 20 minutes of moderate endurance training, there is an increase in natural killer cells (NK) as well as a minor rise in monocytes. The NK cells are not produced in higher numbers, rather larger amounts detach from the internal blood vessel walls. The acting stimulus here is the catecholamine effect which increases cardiac output. After the exertion is over, their number falls to below the original level and remains at a lower level for several hours. The NK cell count rises again at rest and remains constantly elevated in regular moderate-intensity endurance training.

The number of granulocytes, however, does not increase until after a good hour, whereas this increase does then remain constant for another 24 hours and the granulocytes' state of activity is elevated.

The benefits of non-specific immunity are particularly important in old age because they counteract the age-dependent fall in the specific-action T-lymphocytes.

Moderate endurance training is a good immunostimulant.

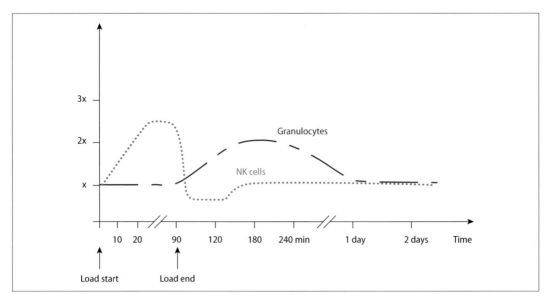

◻ **Fig. 62.1** Cell count changes in moderate endurance workout

63 High-performance sports and non-specific immunity

During strenuous endurance exercises, the secretion of cortisol increases two- to three-fold and then superimposes the effect of the catecholamine release. As a result, the number of NK cells rises up to 9 times the initial value and drops back to 50 % of the initial value for a few hours after exercise has finished. In addition, cytotoxic activity is reduced, regulated by higher prostaglandin F2 levels produced by the monocytes.

Excessive exercise creates an "open window" in the body's immune defenses, making it more vulnerable to pathogens.

Granulocytes behave differently. Their number can increase by up to three times their initial value. Their release from the bone marrow is caused by the cortisol effect. Although they produce 30–50 % fewer **reactive oxygen compounds** under these conditions as a result of their increased numbers, their bactericidal effect is increased overall. These granulocyte changes are reversed after 1–2 days.

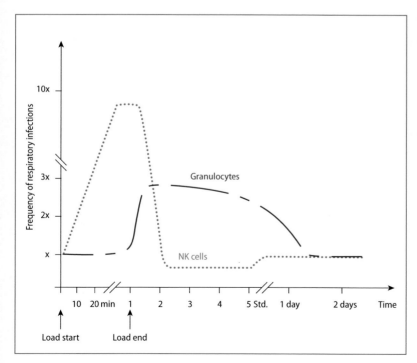

Fig. 63.1 Cell count changes during intensive endurance workout

64 Exercise and optimizing the body's immune defenses

Moderately practiced endurance training in the aerobic range promotes the performance and regeneration capabilities of the immune system.

This lowers infection rates and diminishes the severity of symptoms. A J-shaped correlation exists between endurance training and immunoprotection. Recreational athletes who engage in moderate levels of exercise have the lowest infection risk. Inactivity and more excessive levels of high-performance sports raise the infection risk. In elderly athletes, a weekly regimen of 3–5 hours, distributed over 4–5 training units is ideal. Younger people adapt their immune tolerability to markedly higher aerobic stressors.

Negative changes in the immune defense through occasionally excessive acute physical overexertion are reversible when adequate recovery phases are adhered to. The duration of these phases, however should not be underestimated: after heavy exertion phases, 3–4 days should be allotted for full regeneration. The greater the body's endurance capacity, the better its regeneration capability will be.

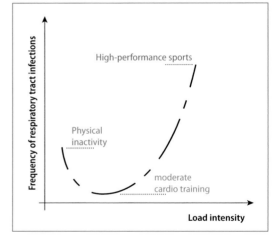

▫ **Fig. 64.1** Amount of physical exercise determines immune protection

Without sufficiently long recovery periods, the immune system will eventually become exhausted.

65 The immunology of overuse syndrome

It is usually inexperienced, overly ambitious athletes who are affected by overuse syndrome. Initially, the afflicted person notices their rapidly waning physical performance capability. Then, health-related impairments develop, the extent of which may be considerable.

Like every physical overload, overtraining syndrome (OTS) starts with an inflammation reaction mediated by the **interleukins 1 and 6** as well as **tumor necrosis factor α** to repair microruptures in muscles and connective tissue. These messenger substances are also produced by the muscles as myokines (▶ Chapter 47).

In the case of chronic physical overloading, the actual local process gradually turns into a systemic one. The **interleukin 1** circulating in the limbic system triggers fatigue and occasional depression. The two interleukins mentioned above cause hormone reductions in the gonads, resulting in irregular menstrual cycles and loss of libido. Moreover, they stimulate the adrenal glands to increase cortisol production. Cortisol promotes the formation of glucose from glutamine. this amino acid is then lacking for special functions in the immune system. In addition, cortisol inhibits **interleukin 2** and thereby negatively impacts the cellular immune defenses.

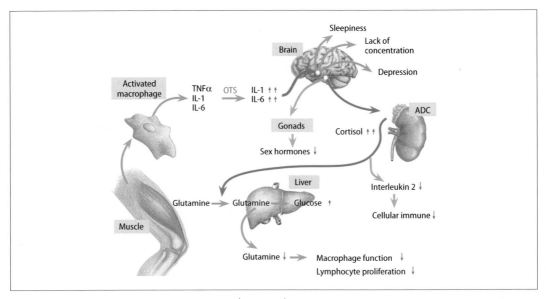

☐ **Fig. 65.1** Biochemical processes during overloading: ↑ increase, ↓ reduction, *OTS* Over Training Syndrome, *ADC* adrenal cortex

66 Endurance training and tumor immunology

The physiological fundamentals known to date suggest that endurance training likely has a positive influence on lowering the risk of malignant diseases. Facts favoring this likelihood include that moderate physical exertion is associated with enhanced mobilization of natural killer cells, their overall higher cytotoxic capacity as well as the phagocytosis capability of granulocytes that is improved under these conditions (▶ Chapter 62). This enables our immune system to attack and eliminate the constant flux of neoplastic cells occurring in our body.

Breast cancer in women is one example of regular physical activity leading to a lower disease incidence and reduced mortality risk. This was shown by the results of 3 large-scaled studies: conducted by the California Teachers Study on more than 130,000, the NIH-AARP Diet and Health study on close to 183,000 and the Nurses' Health Study on over 95,000 participants (Peters et al. 2009, West-Wright et al. 2009, Eliassen et al. 2010). The strongest protection is conferred when physical activity is started at a young age (Maruti et al. 2008, Leitzmann et al. 2008). But even one hour of walking a day reduces the risk of cancer (Hildebrand et al. 2013).

Besides estradiol, insulin also plays a role in the development of breast cancer. This hormone can accelerate the growth of tumor cells. Because overweight persons often have insulin resistance (▶ Chapter 40) and larger concentrations of unbound insulin circulate in their bodies for a period of time, insulin is also a co-factor in the higher rate of breast cancer in obese women. The observed lower frequency of this type of cancer in athletic women is additionally attributable to the weight loss and associated reduction in insulin resistance.

Due to the fact that insulin levels are reduced by endurance training, the risk for bowel cancer is also lower (Wolin et al. 2011). In this context, the authors of this large meta-analysis describe the specific mechanism to be the lower development of adenomas and their slower conversion to malignant carcinoma.

Nevertheless, global protection against malignant tumors by merely strengthening endurance capacity is not tenable given the numerous noxae, developmental mechanisms and, not least, the multitude of individual genetic predispositions that exist. Indeed, any protective effects will only have an impact in the case of very long-term, regular endurance training.

> The significant indirect cancer protection remains unaffected by the direct influence of regular endurance training on preventing malignancy.

Indirect cancer protection can be conferred, e. g., by reducing the proportion of body fat (▶ Chapter 39), improved diet, restraint in alcohol consumption or quitting smoking (Khan et al. 2010, Lee et Derakhshan 2013).

67 Endurance exercise as a rehabilitation intervention after cancer

In the majority of patients, the malignant disease as well as the chemotherapies or radiation treatments required lead to severe **impairment of physical performance** and to **permanent fatigue**. Harmless tasks of everyday life become excruciating burdens – a state that can last for months, sometimes even years. The rapid fatigability enslaves the patient in constant rest. Exercise does not start, if at all, until many weeks after the therapy is over. That means that valuable rehabilitation time is lost.

> Resting is equivalent to a lack of exercise, resulting in muscle atrophy and a further decline in performance capability.

The normal everyday activities become more and more strenuous and the need to recover grows correspondingly larger. Studies have shown, however, that carefully initiated exercise interventions are effective during and absolutely essential after cancer treatments (Brown et al 2011, Rock et al. 2012, Andersen et al. 2013, Wiskemann et Steindorf 2013). Not only are the generally positive effects of endurance training on mind and body even more beneficial for cancer patients earlier on, these patients especially profit from to the rapid **boost to their immune system** that is both crucial to their cure and frequently associated with a reduction in cancer-related mortality.

Carefully dosed muscle-strengthening activities involving all major muscle groups are most suitable for rehabilitation. Training programs should be designed so as to achieve approximately 70 % of maximum achievable load intensity in the end. It is optimal to start with 3 half-hour training units per week, during which frequent breaks are allowed.

After 4–6 weeks, scope and intensity can be increased. Afterwards, the cancer patients may fully exert themselves during their physical activity, at least according to the results of a small, randomized, controlled study on 269 cancer patients of both sexes with a mean age of 47 years (Adamsen et al. 2009). The participants exercised nine hours per week under supervision – half the time at high intensity – and benefitted immensely from their training. Their feeling of permanent fatigue subsided markedly and vitality, emotional well-being, as well as strength and endurance improved significantly compared with a control group. By contrast, such short-term physical activity does not influence general health-related fitness and quality of life (Ballard-Barbash et al. 2012).

68 Speed of energy release I – aerobic muscle endurance

The quality demands placed on the energy supply vary depending on the intensity and duration of the contraction work performed by the muscles. Initially, the phosphate stored in the muscle is available immediately and without oxygen requirement, but is unfortunately only present in low concentrations. The importance of these concentrations is that they more or less instantly enable high performance (► Chapter 6 and ► Chapter 69).

The main energy suppliers are carbohydrates and fats, and proteins to a lesser extent. Since carbohydrate metabolism can be activated considerably faster than fat metabolism, it continually takes precedence and is supplemented in parallel by the initially more sparing energy production from fats. When carbohydrate stores are depleted, the muscles can only work to a limited extent due to the slow glucose neosynthesis in the liver, even though huge energy reserves are stored in the fat depots.

Given sufficient oxygen input, the metabolism of carbohydrates and fats is an **aerobic** process.

However, every kind of aerobic endurance activity starts with oxygen debt because the cardiovascular system and metabolism themselves react to the transition from rest to exercise by increasing their activity levels.

This transition phase takes 2–4 minutes. The oxygen deficit is then compensated for at the end of the exertion by increased oxygen uptake. During physical exertion of low to moderate intensity lasting under one hour, when the cardiovascular system has to provide approximately half its peak performance capability, energy release from carbohydrates and fats takes place in approximately the same proportions. During this process, the measureable activation of fat metabolism is initiated after a delay of 15–30 minutes, depending on the body's fitness level.

When moderate-intensity endurance performance is maintained for over and beyond an hour, the proportion of fat burned in the exerted muscles increases to 60–70 % with equal emptying of the glycogen depots.

69 Speed of energy release II – anaerobic muscle endurance

An increased intensity of exertion goes hand-in-hand with an elevation of energy generation from the carbohydrate metabolism. This does not take place proportionately, but at an over-proportionate ratio to the increase in intensity. The proportion of fat burning decreases correspondingly. Very high intensity exercises can ultimately only be maintained by the carbohydrate metabolism. In this context, the speed of energy provision plays a decisive role. Within an exertion range requiring 50–80 % of the maximum oxygen uptake, the oxygen flooding into the cells takes place fast enough for the carbohydrates to be burned into carbon dioxide and water, i.e. still under aerobic conditions.

However, further increases in the exercise intensities to over 80 % increase the glucose throughput by up to tenfold, i. e., requiring very fast energy flow rates. The amount of transported oxygen per time unit is no longer sufficient for this enormously high glucose breakdown in the active muscle. As a result, the carbohydrates are only broken down incompletely, into lactic acid. Since no oxygen is consumed in this case, we speak of **anaerobic** energy release. This is very inefficient because without oxygen only 5.5 % of the amount of energy is released that might be utilized by a metabolism burning at 100 % efficiency under aerobic conditions.

High-intensity exercise under anaerobic energy generation is possible for approximately 80 seconds. Added to this are around 5 seconds during which energy is taken from the low ATP reserves and around 20 seconds for depleting the creatine phosphate stores. Panic-driven fight-or-flight reactions or the corresponding athletic stressors can thus only be maintained for barely 2 minutes, although the energy stores would be sufficient for 5 minutes under these special conditions. This shortened time is related to a protection mechanism for the muscles. They might become damaged during longer-lasting high-intensity exertion. In order for the body to avoid this, the over-acidification caused by the accumulation of lactic acid in the muscles has a strongly performance-limiting effect. The thus-triggered compulsion to substantially limit or even stop the exercise entirely is usually followed by a more or less rapid recovery phase, depending on the individual's fitness level.

Mostly, the lactate is re-eliminated after 30–60 minutes. The primary sites of lactate metabolism are the liver, heart and skeletal muscle.

70 The myth of effortless fat burning

The concept of moving extremely slowly to burn off as much fat as possible is a commonly practiced ritual among exercise buffs in fitness studios. But such "fat-burning workouts" do not make good physiological sense because carbohydrate metabolism always takes precedence timewise over fat metabolism. The energy equivalent of fatty acids is responsible for their lower energy flow rate. When considered in relation to one liter of oxygen, the energy yield of **fats** is only **4.7 kcal** – despite their more than twice as high energy value – whereas that of **carbohydrates is 5.1 kcal**. The nearly 10 % higher energy generation from carbohydrates and their faster metabolic pathways during the same oxygen consumption are the reasons why the body gives priority to carbohydrates for its energy metabolism.

The process of energy metabolism is extremely complex indeed. It involves energy-rich phosphates like ATP and creatine phosphate, glucose in the blood, glycogen stores in muscles and liver, free fatty acids, triglycerides in the adipose tissue and, in a subordinate role, amino acids from proteins as well. Due to the energy preference towards carbohydrate metabolism, less-fit individuals in particular will mainly burn up the glycogen reserves in their muscles only. Not until they start more intensive training will their metabolism be improved to the extent that their body is also able to intensely mobilize its fat reserves (▶ Chapter 68). The optimal regimen for this is physical exercise in the range of 70 % of the body's peak possible performance.

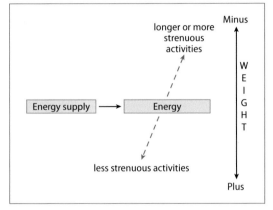

◻ **Fig. 70.1** Effects of energy metabolism on weight

From the perspective of weight loss, success or failure are dictated entirely by the laws of physics: **the principle of conservation of energy** formulated by Robert Mayer back in 1842. According to this principle, you can only reduce your weight while maintaining the same energy input by increasing your energy output.

The more strenuous physical activity is, the more negative the energy balance and, consequently, the greater the weight loss from fat metabolism.

71 Endurance training and temperature regulation

Physical performance is always associated with increased heat generation. This is because the chemical energy of nutrients can only be converted into work output at an efficiency rate of around 40 % (▶ Chapter 6). Since our survival depends on us living within a temperature-controlled range, any excess heat generated must immediately be channeled off. During strenuous physical exertion or at high ambient temperatures, radiation or convection play only minor roles. Much more important for this process are the dilated vessels and **sweat production** followed by evaporative cooling. Under these circumstances, the latter constitutes up to 70 % of our heat dissipation. We can produce from 1–2 liters of sweat per hour, in extreme situations as much as 2.5 liters. Approximately half of the sweat produced evaporates off, extracting heat from the body in the magnitude of 575 kcal per liter in dry to moderately humid air. For example, the energy expenditure of a person weighing 70 kg during a one-hour run over 10 km is approximately 700 kcal, meaning that approx. 420 kcal fall to heat development. On a sunny day between spring and fall, one-third of this amount of energy is added in the form of absorbed sunlight, making it necessary to dissipate nearly 575 kcal of heat in this scenario. That equates to the evaporative cooling of around one liter of sweat.

The body can tolerate minor losses of fluids without problems. However, under intensive exertion, when sweat production is very high, one of the measurable effects of this is a reduction in the circulating blood volume. That causes the heart beat

volume to drop, the body to initiate compensatory reactions with an increased heart rate. To achieve optimal thermoregulation, i. e., transfer heat from inside to outside the body, the vessels of the skin show a reflex response called vasodilation, wherein the effective blood volume is lowered even further. Before these various mechanisms cause heat damage, the body's performance capability is initially reduced. This becomes noticeable even if the reduction in flowing blood volume is only around 3 %, or approximately 150–180 ml.

> As a rule of thumb for calculating the effect of overall fluid loss: performance losses of 10 % can be expected for every 1 % of body weight fluid lost.

When compensating for lost water volume, consider the fact that around 40 % of the water volume excreted through the sweat over one hour of endurance training derives from metabolic processes and therefore does not need to be replenished immediately. Therefore, it is sufficient to drink half to one liter of fluids at the most per hour of normal-intensity endurance training at outdoor temperatures. If the body is pumped with too much fluid, there is a short term elevation in blood volume and, as a consequence, a relative fall in electrolyte levels. The thereby lowered salt concentrations caused by the very high-volume **fluid overload** can induce states of confusion or seizures.

72 The biomechanics of running

Barefoot or minimally shod runners tend to land on the fore- or mid-foot. In contrast, the running shoes popular today, with their elevated and cushioned heels, tend to cause many joggers to rear-foot strike, thereby exposing them to a higher incidence of repetitive stress injuries (Lieberman et al. 2010). As a result of this cushioning, the collision forces exerted on the forefoot are lower than on the heel.

> The basic skeletal structure of the foot is made up of 26 bones, with a total of 45 muscles per leg necessary to carry the body and ensure the body's locomotion in its upright position.

During locomotion, the feet must absorb two force peaks per step: a shock-absorbing impact peak approximately 20-30 milliseconds (ms) after ground contact and a push-off peak after a further 70 ms that again propels the foot in the direction of walking. In the push-off phase, the bone and joint stresses are higher than during the foot-strike phase. During a normal landing phase, the foot initially contacts the ground with its front outer edge, then rolls inwardly and pronates during a very short stance phase.

The stresses exerted on the lower extremities during this phase are tremendous. Depending on the speed of locomotion, each step causes the ankle joint to be subject to 2.2 to 4.8 times the body's weight for 20-40 ms. On average, the weight-bearing stresses for a person weighing 75 kg running a distance of 1 kilometer (1200 steps) add up to around 160 tons spread over 18 seconds for each foot.

In other words, those individuals who, in addition to their daily walking distances, do 20 km per week of jogging over a period of 40 years will have subjected each ankle to about 6.5 million tons of stress spread over about 200 hours. This load-withstanding feat demonstrates the amazing adaptability of biological tissues. The training effect on muscle growth, in particular, is measurable just a few weeks after beginning an exercise regimen or increasing the scope of training activities (▶ Chapter 79). Connective tissue, however, does not behave quite as effectively during these adaptation processes. Because of their lower metabolic activity, structures such as cartilage, tendons, ligaments and capsules need up to 12 months to adapt.

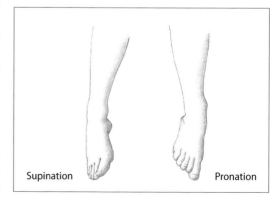

Supination   Pronation

☐ **Fig. 72.1** Load-bearing foot postures (exaggerated representation)

73 Required features for running shoes

The enormous stresses put on joints, muscles and connective tissues during locomotion demonstrate the paramount importance of proper footwear. Improper footwear can quickly cause discomfort, in the same way that a change of running shoes can work wonders for those who experience running-related pain. Unfortunately, there is no one-size-fits-all shoe that is "right" for every type of runner. Individual body weight, malpositioning of the feet or legs and incorrect foot alignment are just a few examples of why runners must always personalize their choice of footwear. Basically, a running shoe should interfere as little as possible with the foot's natural kinematic processes. Flexible soles ensure optimal rolling (heel-to-toe movement) of the shoe and thus effective force transmission from foot to ground. Stiff soles, on the other hand, force the foot into a levering motion and can cause overuse injuries because more work is transferred to the toes.

Soles and heels of running shoes should not be too thick or too wide because they intensify the effect of uneven terrain and increase the risk of twisting an ankle. Thick soles also put undue stress on the Achilles tendon because they create greater leverage forces when the foot hits the ground during laterally directed heel-to-toe movement. Light-weight footwear can force the supporting muscles to work harder in untrained individuals. Because they offer more support, firmer shoes are more appropriate for beginners.

If this "wiggle room" is missing, long periods of exercise can result in painful toenails with bruising underneath as well as the associated cramped running style. Running shoes should also feature customizable lacing. Too-loose laces are often the cause of knee pain and shin splints due to heel slippage. On the other hand, very painful pressure symptoms can occur when the lacing over the upper bridge of the foot is drawn too tight in individuals with high arches. It makes sense for runners with extensive workout routines to switch shoes regularly. This will vary, and thereby partially alleviate, the stresses exerted on joints and muscles.

The use of prescription orthopedic insoles for the acute treatment of overuse injuries should be reviewed at intervals of several weeks to several months because the insoles themselves can cause overuse injuries due to changes in foot biomechanics. It must also be remembered that the lower extremities are subject to immense stress just by normal everyday life. That is how street shoes worn every day can also cause overuse injuries. However, this fact usually escapes the attention of those afflicted because they usually do not notice the pain until greater forces are applied during exercise, leading the wearer to mistakenly blame their running shoes.

When purchasing running shoes, take into consideration that the shoe shortens during heel-to-toe movements. Therefore, the toes should have about 10 mm of "wiggle room" at the front.

74 Physical exercise and the skeletal system

The major positive effects of strength and endurance training on bones and joints include:
- increase in bone mass
- increase in cartilage metabolism
- cross-sectional enlargement of the fibrils in connective tissue structures

The supporting tissue in the human body includes approximately 208 bones, the number of which can vary slightly from individual to individual. The bones make up 12–14 % of the body's weight.

The most common cells in bone are **osteocytes**. Osteocytes are former osteoblasts that have become permanently embedded within the bone matrix after fulfilling their function of building up bone. The long-living osteocytes send out signals telling the body where and how much bone needs to be renewed by **osteoclasts** and **osteoblasts**.

The sum of all forces working on the bone dictates the degree of cellular activity in the bone. That is also how proper exercise stimuli can achieve a measurable gain in bone mass (▶ Chapter 77). However, only skeletal portions affected by muscle contraction forces respond to these stimuli. Stress stimuli must significantly exceed those of normal daily activities.

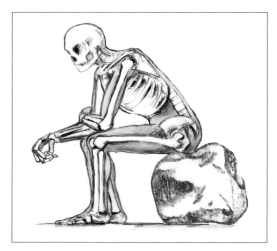

◘ **Fig. 74.1** A skeleton taking a break

A large amount of muscle mass usually correlates with healthy bone strength.

An increase in bone mass of up to 1 % per year is possible. this is identical to the natural rate of decrease in bone mass starting at about the age of 35.

75 The constant renewal of bone

Bone is a highly metabolically active tissue. The biochemical processes that take place in bone are all aimed at maintaining an adequate organic matrix and normal mineralization thereof. **Collagen** comprises 90 % of the protein matrix of bone, **osteocalcin** and several other proteins make up the other 10 %. **Mineralization** occurs mainly by incorporation of **calcium salts**, which give bone its stability.

The breakdown and build-up of bone are tightly coupled and both form part of the process of bone remodeling, an active and dynamic process that takes place continually throughout an individual's lifetime. 1.5 million such processes are constantly undergoing different phases in the skeleton. Repair mechanisms take 90–100 days to complete. 25 % of trabecular bone, e. g. in the vertebral bodies, renews itself per year, but only 3 % of the outer shell of long bones. If the degradation of bone exceeds that of bone formation over a longer period, **osteoporosis** is the result.

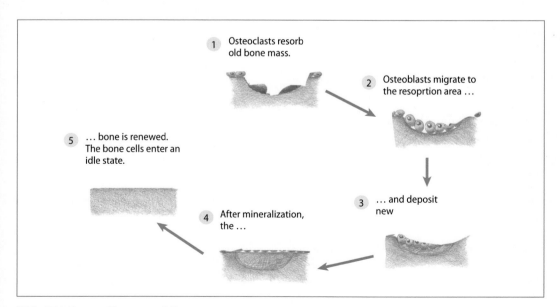

1 Osteoclasts resorb old bone mass.

2 Osteoblasts migrate to the resoprtion area …

5 … bone is renewed. The bone cells enter an idle state.

3 … and deposit new

4 After mineralization, the …

◻ **Fig. 75.1** Process of bone remodeling

76 Osteoporosis

An important regulator of the constant process of bone formation and resorption is the RANKL/RANK system. This control loop is disrupted in osteoporosis. Osteoporosis is a systemic skeletal disease characterized by low bone mass and impaired microarchitecture of bony tissue (Baum et Peters 2008, Compston et al. 2013). The receptor activator of nuclear factor kappa-B ligands (**RANKL**) also appears to regulate temperature rises to fight off infection with RANK docking molecules (Hanada et al. 2009).

Humans with healthy bones reach their maximum bone mass density in life in early adulthood, around age 20–25. Bone mass density is especially high in individuals who follow a diet rich in calcium and vitamin D3, get regular sun exposure and exercise frequently. With increasing age, the risk of developing osteoporosis also increases considerably. Other risk factors include genetic predisposition, sedentary lifestyle, low-calcium diet, high protein and phosphate intake, nicotine or alcohol abuse, underweight (Compston et al. 2014), early menopause (in women) or medications such as glucocorticoids, laxatives, anti-epileptic drugs and thyroid hormones.

Reduced bone strength can quickly turn slight injuries into bone fractures. At a substance loss of 40 %, this affects one in two individuals. Almost any kind of fracture is possible. In 2009, 5.2 million women and 1.1 million men in Germany were stricken by osteoporosis (Hadji et al. 2013). This

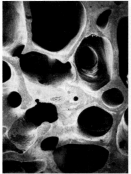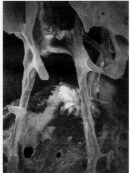

◘ Fig. 76.1 Bone structure: Left: normal structure, right: Osteoporosis

study estimated that around 885,000 cases are newly diagnosed every year. Every year in that country, about 110,000 people with this degenerative disease suffer a hip fracture. about 30 % of them die within a year and another 30 % are permanently incapacitated.

Homocysteine impairs the stabilizing matrix of collagen fibrils in the skeletal system by means of short-chain crosslinks (van Wijngaarden et al. 2013).

> In patients with osteoporosis, high homocysteine levels are associated with an increased fracture rate.

77 Strength training

Strength and (to a lesser extent) endurance training lead to muscle growth and strength gains.
   Strength training
- stabilizes bone and joints,
- lowers the risk of osteoporosis,
- and accelerates the basal metabolic rate, consequently resulting in weight loss and optimized metabolism.

The strength of the skeletal muscles in humans reaches their individual peak at approximately age 23. In women, these muscles make up about 30 % of body weight and in men 40 %. In physically inactive individuals, muscle mass decreases gradually up to the age of 55 and then at an accelerated pace, whereby the lower extremities are usually affected to a greater degree. By the age of 75, the overall muscle loss can reach 25–35 %.

> Muscle breakdown causes an unfavorable shift in the power-to-weight ratio.

Joints, ligaments and tendons are no longer relieved by strong muscles. This disproportion between load and load-bearing capacity elevates the risk of falls and injuries, making limitations in the activities of daily life commonplace. A regular and varied training regimen, however, can keep physical strength and bone density at a nearly youthful level. The

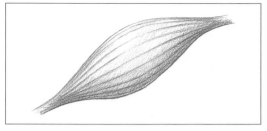

▢ Fig. 77.1

several hundred skeletal muscles put into action for this can be trained well into old age.
   But muscles are not just working machines. This becomes clear when looking at the fiber composition of muscle nerves. Less than 20 % of nerve fibers are intended for motor tasks. By contrast, a good 80 % of the fibers are made up of approximately 50 % vasomotor and 50 % sensory portions (Leyk 2009). Even during short periods of loading, vasomotor fibers ensure an immediate increase in local blood circulation in the muscles and thus contribute to strengthening the cardiovascular system. The sensory fibers of muscle nerves react in a very sophisticated manner. They influence important control systems in the body via a complex interlinking with the central nervous system. Not least, muscles produce a wealth of important chemicals critical to metabolic processes (▶ Chapter 47). Precisely this fact provides an additional explanation for the positive effects of exercise on both psyche and immune system.

78 Potential muscle stressors

Most muscles are designed to work in functional pairs. When a muscle is flexed by the **agonist**, its counterpart or **antagonist** can counter act this flexion by extending the muscle again. The local force exerted by the neuromuscular system depends on the number, cross-section and structure of the individual muscle fibers. Optimal coordination of the respective cooperating muscles and the efficient provision of energy also play an important role.

Muscles can be exerted in a great multitude of different ways. For example, during the **development of dynamic forces** within a sequence of movements, the emphasis is on shortening of the muscles, also known as **concentric contraction** (i.e., muscle contraction in which the ends of the muscle move together towards a common center). When the application of force against resistance lengthens the muscle, e.g. like the braking force necessary to walk

downhill or the body bracing itself after raising a weight, this is known as **eccentric work** (elongation of the fibers back out from a common center). If the contraction is directed against insurmountable resistance, this is a **static strength exercise**. During this **isometric muscle tensioning**, muscle length remains unchanged. A muscle's maximum eccentric strength is always greater than its dynamic maximum strength, and, depending on training status, 5–40 % greater than its static strength.

In terms of sport or exercise, we are usually dealing with dynamic forces. The sequence of movements during running, for example, but also in many other sports, is characterized by rhythmic alternation between concentric contraction and eccentric braking force. The contraction velocity dictates the performance of the related muscles.

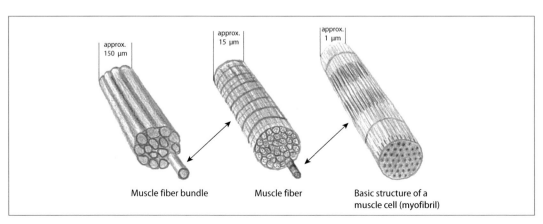

approx. 150 µm

approx. 15 µm

approx. 1 µm

Muscle fiber bundle   Muscle fiber   Basic structure of a muscle cell (myofibril)

◘ **Fig. 78.1** Structure of fasciated muscle

79 Increasing muscular endurance

A well-balanced muscle training program should be carried out 2 to 4 times a week and be based on the loads demanded during sports and everyday activities. Between 3 and 5 sets of each exercise should be carried out. The type and order of the exercises should be continually varied to set new training incentives. In this regard, it is advisable to only moderately increase the scope and intensity of the exercises. If you train on consecutive days, be sure to work different muscle groups than those worked the previous day. To prevent acute injuries, exercises must be carried out slowly and at a steady pace. Jerky movements can very quickly damage muscles and connective tissue.

Slow motion phases are also optimal for increasing strength. Lifting and lowering a weight and the pause in between repetitions should likewise each last roughly 2 seconds. These exercises should result in significant fatigue of the exerted muscles. To protect the spine, avoid hunching over or rounding your back. Exhale when raising the weight and inhale when lowering it. when performing isometric exercises, take short, quick breaths. Holding your breath is never a good idea. 1–2 minutes of rest should be taken between sets.

The first signs of progress can be seen after about 3 weeks and are mainly due to an improvement in neuromuscular coordination. Muscle

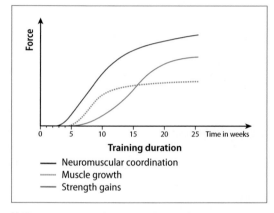

■ **Fig. 79.1** Training duration and strength gains

growth generally begins after 4–6 weeks and is associated with a gain in strength.

> The slower the gain in strength, the more slowly strength is lost during periods of physical inactivity.

One workout a week is generally enough to maintain strength.

80 Weight gain due to muscle atrophy

Muscle atrophy due to physical inactivity (► Chapter 77) not only makes us lethargic and potentially ill, it also makes us fat. The following **sample calculation** demonstrates this:

In a young men, the proportion of muscle mass in relation to body weight should be around 40 %. A man with a total body weight of 75 kg theoretically should have 30 kg of muscle. This muscle mass alone is responsible for a daily energy consumption of approx. 450 kcal at the basal metabolic rate (2700 kcal total energy expenditure, two-thirds of which or 1800 kcal are burned by the basal metabolism, one-quarter of them utilized by the muscles). Accordingly, a kilogram of muscle built by training burns about 15 kcal a day even at rest: That corresponds to a weight of 650 g of fat per year. This calculation takes into account that fatty tissue binds around 10 % water. Conversely, every kilogram of muscle mass lost every year leaves a considerable amount of fat untouched in the subcutaneous compartments, which then expand more and more with increasing age. Within 10 years, that would translate into a weight gain of 6.5 kg under otherwise identical living conditions.

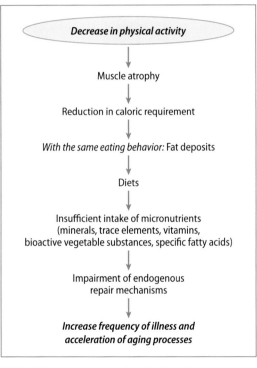

□ **Fig. 80.1** Consequences of physical inactivity

The more muscle mass that can be mobilized during physical activity, the greater is the energy expenditure and the more adipose tissue melts off.

The active metabolic rate benefits from muscle buildup as well. Thus, because younger athletes are usually equipped with more muscle mass than older ones, they usually don't have to exercise as much as older ones to lose the same amount of weight.

81 Muscular imbalances

From an evolutionary perspective, muscles can be categorized as phasic, tonic or mixed. Purely phasic muscles were originally responsible for movement and tend to weaken. Tonic muscles developed to perform static work and tend to shorten. Today, the mixed form is found in human skeletal muscle (◻ Tab. 81.1).

Depending on which specific type of fiber predominates, muscles are classified as more phasic or more tonic. Routine improper loads and one-sided training stimuli, where injuries are often a causal co-factor, can easily lead to muscular imbalances.

Although it is always useful to strengthen and stretch as many muscles as possible to keep the body healthy, the particulars of the different fiber types must be taken into account when there are muscular imbalances. In this case, the phasic muscles, with a tendency to weaken, should be strengthened, while stretching should take priority for the tonic muscles.

◻ **Tab. 81.1** Reaction of important muscles to improper stresses/loading in physical activity (▶ Figure 82.1).

Tend to weaken (phasic muscles)	Tend to shorten (tonic muscles)
1 Rhomboid muscles	10 Levator scapulae muscle
2 Ascending and transverse trapezius	11 Descending trapezius
3 Triceps brachii muscle	12 Pectoralis major muscle
4 Central part of the latissimus dorsi muscle	13 Biceps brachii muscle
5 Rectus abdominis muscle latissimus dorsi muscle	14 Upper and lower part of the latissimus dorsi muscle
6 Gluteal muscles (gluteus maximus, medius, minimus)	15 Iliopsoas
7 Vastus lateralis muscle A and vastus medialis muscles B	16 Gracilis muscle
	17 Rectus femoris muscle
8 Tibialis anterior muscle	18 Adductor brevis, longus, magnus muscles)
9 Peronei muscles	19 Piriformis muscle
	20 Semimembranosus muscle A, semitendinosus muscle B, biceps femoris muscle C
	21 Gastrocnemius muscle A, soleus muscle B

82 Precautionary measures during strength training

Extreme exertion may not always be without health risks. The main reason for this is the tendency to hold one's breath during lifts when working with heavy weights. When exhaling forcibly against a closed glottis like this (called a Valsalva maneuver), elevated pressures of 100–200 mmHg build up in the chest cavity. Indeed, the spine is stabilized by this, providing the muscles with a firmer structural basis. At the same time, however, internal veins are constricted and neck and forehead veins heavily congested. The face turns red as a sign of rising blood pressure. Strength exercises involving the arms lead to higher amplitudes than those using the legs. These processes are not dangerous for healthy people. In risk persons with a previously damaged cardiovascular system, however, they can cause cardiac arrhythmia or stroke. A sports physician's advice is compulsory for these persons before starting a strength training program.

For the elderly, it is advisable to always perform strength training with larger muscle groups in a very controlled manner and with a limited number of sets. Resistance exercises should be limited to about 50 % of maximum strength. When performed regularly, resistance training like this can even permanently lower blood pressure in a similar magnitude to endurance training (▶ Chapter 53).

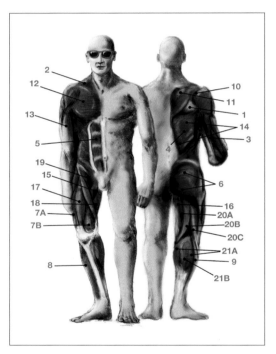

◻ **Fig. 82.1** Anatomy of important muscles in the musculoskeletal system (see also ◻ Tab. 81.1)

83 Mobility Exercises

Mobility is determined by two factors, **flexibility** and **elasticity**. The individual characteristics of the joints and intervertebral discs are responsible for the former and the muscles, ligaments and tendons for the latter. Children generally have very good mobility, but unless it is trained, it becomes distinctly limited even in adolescents and further decreases with age. Women are usually more flexible than men because of their slightly lower muscle mass. Good mobility translates into an optimal ability to relax the muscles. Stress tolerance increases as well. Strength and agility should be trained in parallel where possible.

After strenuous exercise, careful stretching can bring tired, shortened muscles back to their normal length. During **static stretching**, the muscles are stretched as far as possible and held in this position over 20–60 seconds. **Dynamic stretching** is essentially rhythmic stretching, e.g. performing rocking movements to stretch the calf muscles. All stretches should be pain-free. Recently injured muscles must not be stretched.

Regular flexibility training in non-athletic adults is mainly aimed at mobility maintenance and less on improving mobility. The result is a reduced

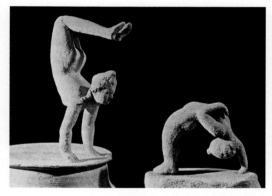

◩ **Fig. 83.1** Hippocrates had already stressed the importance of gymnastics for preserving health. (Courtesy of Andreas Verlag, Salzburg)

tendency to fall and in old age and thus fewer bone fractures in those with existing osteoporosis.

> At any age, flexibility training plays an important role in protecting against acute injuries and chronic overuse damage.

84 Balance training

A good sense of balance is essential for proper spatial orientation and posture. Younger people generally have an excellent sense of balance. By contrast, aging is usually characterized by weight gain and a loss of balance. Regular balance exercises therefore make sense at any age, but they are of particularly high importance for older people (Clemson et al. 2012). Regularly practicing mobility also enhances coordination and the diversity of autonomous movement patterns. Accidents due to clumsiness can be avoided entirely or dealt with more successfully. Numerous sports demonstrate the importance of optimal equilibrium training.

> Well-tuned interaction between the various muscle groups and the central nervous system also translates into a reduction in the oxygen and energy the body requires, as well as optimization of movement sequences.

For elderly people, simple but efficient balance exercises are recommended. These should consist of daily practice standing on one leg while donning and doffing socks and shoes without leaning against any objects.

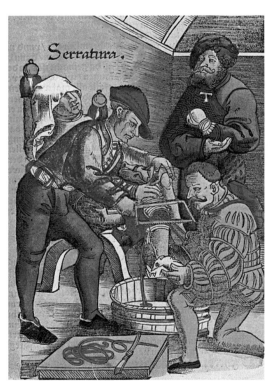

◘ **Fig. 84.1** Leg amputation, Xylograph by J. Wetchlin (1540). (Courtesy of Andreas Verlag, Salzburg)

85 Sitting too much leads to an early grave

The previous chapters illustrated the positive health-related effects that can be achieved through regular physical activity. Endurance training is especially health-promoting and life-prolonging (Schnohr et al. 2013). More strenuous physical activities increase the health effect. This has been confirmed, among others, by the results of a large study on 654,827 people (Moore et al. 2012). Physical activity from early adolescence on is best (Ekelund et al. 2012). That is why it is very important to help younger people establish healthy habits early on. However, even physical stressors after years of inactivity improve the chances of reaching a higher age.

It's never too late to start exercising.

Unfortunately, the majority of adults do not engage in regular physical exercise and thus do not reap the associated benefits. Instead, most of them have an additional problem they might not even be aware of: **They sit too much.**

Our early ancestors were hunter-gatherers who traveled 20-30 km daily to procure the food necessary to survive. 100 years ago, the rural population still walked 10-20 km every day. the daily walking distance of the today's Homo sapiens is limited to about 600 m. Instead of walking, we now sit constantly: at the table at dinner, in our cars on the way to work, in the office and in front of the omnipresent TV. Our changing industrial society and the social environment that comes with it have created these conditions. But continuous sitting is a pathogenic risk factor. Less calories are burned, which leads to weight gain, often causing poor spinal posture and thus chronic back pain. Ultimately, the skeletal muscles are generally weakened as well. Prolonged sitting is particularly damaging to blood vessels, increasing the risk of cardiovascular disease. Sitting has always been the unhealthiest posture in humans. The WHO recommends that this posture be limited to 8 hours a day, i.e. that people should stand up as often as possible.

In one large Australian study, 22,497 adults aged over 44 were observed for about 5 years (van der Ploeg et al. 2012). During this period, 5,405 people died. The longer the daily sedentary time, the higher the mortality risk. This special relationship between mortality risk and time spent sitting is true even for those who exercise regularly, albeit to a lesser extent. This comes as no surprise, given that people who are physically active for half an hour a day can still spend about 14 waking hours per day sitting. A large meta-analysis of data on 794,577 persons showed that very long periods of sitting not only trigger cardiovascular diseases, but also significantly increases the risk for type 2 diabetes (Wilmot et al. 2012) and various cancers, such as colon cancer or lung cancer (Schmid et Leitzmann 2014).

86 "Sports are murderous" or sudden cardiac death

It is not clear whether Winston Churchill really said "First of all, no sports" in response to the question as to how he had reached such an advanced age. The phrase became coined in German "Sports are murderous" and erroneously attributed to Churchill's wicked wit. Irrespective of who this quote is attributed to, sports-related deaths are indeed an unfortunate reality.

They occur most frequently in soccer, followed by cycling, jogging and swimming. In an older retrospective study of 29,436 victims over a period of 30 years, 95 % of the deceased men had a mean age of 54 years. These athletes were certainly not healthy, but the crux of the problem is that the athletes at risk are often unaware of their serious diseases. Cardiomyopathy, for example, which is generally inherited, is the most common cause of sudden cardiac death among 20- to 30-year-old men, and coronary heart disease among athletes over 40 years of age. However, inflammation of the heart muscle (myocarditis) and the endocardium (endocarditis) are also frequently the cause of fatal events. The fatal symptom of these inflammatory diseases is uncorrectable arrhythmia. According to reports from the International Olympic Committee, 2 out of every 100,000 physically active people between 12 and 35 years of age die of sudden cardiac death annually. In the non-athletic population, this figure is only 0.7 in 100,000. Sudden cardiac death incidence during physical activity is much higher in men than in women (Marijon et al. 2013). Getting regularly medical screening exams is therefore obligatory for athletes (▶ Chapter 89).

Sudden death from exercise is an omnipresent risk. That said, people are mere mortals. They can die everywhere and at all kinds of occasions. Most frequently, death happens in bed, but also when engaging in physical activity. However, it is very rare that the exercise led to their death.

Life-threatening cardiac arrhythmias can also occur without any serious underlying disease. High-intensity endurance training namely is associated with general vasodilation of the venous vessels in the working muscles. This adaptation is the body's way of optimizing heat dissipation. When endurance activity is terminated abruptly, the circulation is deprived for a few minutes of a certain amount of the blood needed to fill up the additional vessel volume created by vasodilation and the blood pressure drops as a consequence. The body attempts to counteract this reaction by increasing the secretion of vasoconstricting catecholamines. However, higher levels of catecholamines can also induce cardiac arrhythmias. The associated risk increases significantly in conjunction with a drop in blood pressure. To avoid serious incidents, individuals engaging in exercise should therefore gradually decrease the intensity after heavy endurance training, or at least "walk it off," or, if that is no longer possible due to extreme exhaustion, then lie down.

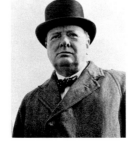

☐ **Fig. 86.1** Winston Churchill (1874–1965). (From: United Nations Information Office, New York [Public domain], courtesy of Wikimedia Commons)

87 Sports injuries and pain defense

Our bodies have special sensory pain receptors that can recognize impending or existing tissue damage. These **nociceptors** are located at the ends of the thin A and C fibers in all organs except for the central nervous system. Pain stimuli first travel through these fibers to the **wide dynamic range neurons (WDRs)** in the dorsal horn of the spinal cord where they are then transmitted to the brain via intermediate-type neurons called interneurons. This is where the first sensory perception of "pain" arises. If the pain goes untreated, the **WDRs** are triggered by the constant firing of impulses and the processes described escalate. The conduction of pain signals is multiplied by the formation of new receptors and ion channels. Previously low-threshold action potentials are now registered by the brain and even spontaneous discharges by these nerve cells are possible without receiving pain signals from the affected nociceptors. All of this triggers enhanced pain perception.

> Fortunately, humans are equipped with a very effective endogenous pain defense system.

The brain stem releases special messenger substances (neurotransmitters) and opioids which significantly limit the action of the pain-transmitting WDRs. One important task in pain defense is the responsibility of the nerve cells to perform a blocking function within this chain of events. The nerve cells are the antagonists of the pain neurons and are interconnected between them. They are also activated with every acute pain trigger and thereby down-regulate overreactions in the pain-processing centers.

> Physical activity promotes the function of pain-inhibiting nerve cells.

Unfortunately, when the pain stimuli persist, the mechanisms of pain inhibition frequently fail. Then, the risk of the pain becoming chronic increases as the body develops a **pain memory**. People with headaches and back problems are most commonly affected by this phenomenon. Fast and long-lasting pain control is therefore always a high priority.

The treatment of sports injuries thus requires very careful attention. As active physical movements effectively support pain control, regenerative training should be initiated as early as possible. Over-ambitious training should certainly be avoided under these circumstances because residual pain can easily cause wrong motion patterns which often lead to a muscular dysbalance which, in turn, can trigger recurrent pain.

88 Sore muscles

After unaccustomed or comparatively intensive physical exercise, pain frequently develops in the muscles made to work. The affected muscles are perceived as weak, hard and tender to the touch. Tears in parts of the muscle fibers, especially in the Z-bands, are thought to be a cause for sore muscles (formerly called muscle catarrh).

Water slowly seeps into the slightly damaged muscle fibers, which swell up and stretch, thereby triggering pain. In addition, this stretching constricts the blood vessels and impairs circulation, thereby intensifying the pain even further. That is why it takes 1–3 days until the pain sensation reaches its peak and then gradually subsides again. Sterile inflammation arises as a consequence of the traumatized fibers breaking down. The unfolding repair mechanisms leave behind a somewhat stronger muscle. After approximately 3 higher-intensity training sessions, the affected muscle adapts to its new demands and no further soreness is experienced.

As muscle fibers produce the greatest forces during eccentric contractions, it is this type of loading that most frequently causes sore muscles (▶ Chapter 78). Sore muscles do not leave any permanent damage behind and the soreness cannot be re-triggered by performing the same movements over several weeks. Careful stretching and mild dynamic movements can help resolve these symptoms. Visits to the sauna or warm baths can also provide some relief. There is no miracle cure that can make sore muscles go away faster. The soreness disappears by itself after 3–4 days.

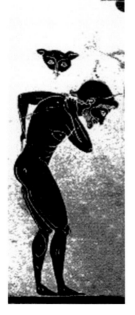

◻ **Fig. 88.1** A man taking a cold shower after physical exercise – as Hippocrates recommended (around 300 BC). (Courtesy of Andreas Verlag, Salzburg)

89 Sports medicine screening examinations

Medical screening by a sports physician is necessary to prevent physical activity from damaging health and is highly advisable
- from the age of 35 years, after longer periods of physical inactivity,
- in apparently healthy persons with one or more risk factors,
- after recovery from any serious illness.

The medical screening examination by a sports physician should cover the patient's general and exercise-related medical history, including a physical examination at the least. Special attention should be paid to any increased risk for cardiovascular diseases. Patients with serious acute or chronic diseases, regardless of the cause, should avoid sports. Over-ambitious athletes, determined to achieve their sporting goals at all costs, are more likely to ignore common sense when suffering from a febrile infection.

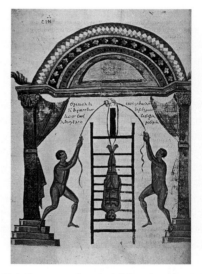

◘ Fig. 89.1 Treatment of a spinal dislocation. (courtesy of Andreas Verlag, Salzburg)

> Fever, however, is an absolute contraindication to engaging in physical activities.

Mild chronic diseases or congenital organic impairments often dictate the necessary limitations. Anyone known to have such health-related disorders should discuss with their doctor whether or not physical exertion is advisable. If so, a personalized training regimen, adapted to the person's physical circumstances, should be developed in consultation with a sports physician. As studies on exercise ther-apy have shown, patients usually benefit greatly by participating in competently supervised sports rehabilitation programs for cardiovascular diseases, cancer or diseases of the musculoskeletal system (Chiaranda et al. 2013).

One special parameter of screening programs for persons over 65 years of age is to measure their treadmill walking speed. The faster they can walk, the fitter and stronger they are, and the longer they tend to live as well. These are the findings based on data from 9 cohort studies on over 34,000 persons and observation periods of between 6 and 21 years (Studenski et al. 2011).

90 Physical activity and air pollution – fine particulate matter

The main causes of outdoor air pollution are industrial complexes, automotive traffic, power stations and waste incineration plants. Indoor air pollution is commonly due to outdated wood-burning fireplaces and the regular use of candles in poorly ventilated rooms.

Particulate matter with a particle size less than 10 μm (PM_{10}) is absorbed by the lungs and can accumulate into an average absorption of 5–7 g per year. In comparison: a human hair has a diameter of 40–100 μm. The minute trace particles of 1–2.5 μm in size are particularly insidious because they can reach the alveoli in the lungs. Although these fine particles are broken down there, the elimination process can take several months. While there, this **fine particulate matter** triggers increased secretion of pro-inflammatory messenger substances. That is how they hasten the progression of atherosclerotic processes (Adar et al. 2013) as well as causing chronic changes in the respiratory tract. In the worst cases, this condition can progress to asthma or even lung cancer (Chen et Goldberg 2009, Andersen et al. 2011, Raaschou-Nielsen et al. 2013).

Ultrafine particles measuring less than 1 μm in diameter can penetrate the wall of the alveoli and migrate into the bloodstream. These particles can cause cardiac arrhythmias and promote the formation of clots by stimulating platelet function, in turn elevating the risk for myocardial infarction or stroke (Tonne et Wilkinson 2013, Shah et al. 2013). The nervous system may also be harmed by impaired brain function. with the elderly and children being particularly susceptible. Mortality is increased across Europe (Beelen et al. 2014). The German

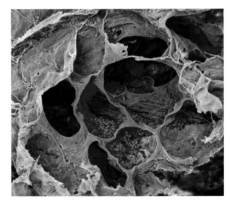

◻ **Fig. 90.1** Image using a scanning electron microscope (SEM). View into the lung with alveoli cut open to expose accumulated red blood cells. (courtesy of Photou. Presse-agentur GmbH FOCUS, Hamburg)

Environmental Protection Agency estimated (2013) that air pollution from fine dust particles is responsible for approximately 47,000 premature deaths every year in Germany alone.

There does not appear to be a risk-free minimum concentration of dust particles. The EU Directive defined levels of 25 μg per cubic meter of air in 24 hours as a compromise from a medically reasonable and technically achievable perspective. This should not be exceeded more than 35 times per year. Exercise and sports on roads with a high volume of traffic is to be avoided.

91 Exercise and air pollution – ozone

A high volume of automotive traffic is responsible for an increased concentration of near-ground **ozone**. An ozone layer cannot form without nitric oxides, up to 70 % of which comes from the combustion processes that run motor vehicles. When the sun goes down, the weaker solar radiation causes the ozone molecules to break down quickly as part of a reverse reaction, provided nitric oxides from car emissions are available as reactants in this process.

Normally in the summer, ozone concentrations are at harmless levels of about 30 µg per m³ of air in populous urban areas. Even short periods of ozone levels of up to 180 µg/m³ do not pose a health risk for the majority of the population. However, sensitivity to ozone varies greatly among individuals. Some people are affected by values as low as 180 µg/m³ under, even if they are only exposed for a few hours. Clinical symptoms include headaches, coughing, breathing problems, fatigue or rapid, shallow breathing under exertion. There is an absolute danger to health involving the compromise of the cellular immune defense or loss of lung tissue elasticity when a person is exposed to a mean level of 360 µg/m³ (EU warning level) for one hour and longer.

When ozone reacts with fine particulate matter, energy-rich oxygen compounds are formed for several seconds that, in turn, cause pollen to become more allergenic and increase the frequency and severity of allergies (Shiraiwa et al. 2011, Beck et al. 2013). In addition, ozone can destroy the cilia of the respiratory tract, causing an accumulation of foreign bodies in the lung. According to data from

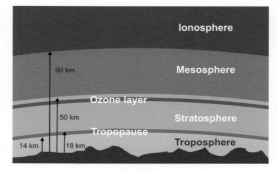

□ **Fig. 91.1** Structure of the atmosphere

a large-scale American study, people who live permanently in areas with high ozone levels have a 3 times higher risk of death caused by respiratory diseases (Jerrett et al. 2009).

> On hot summer days, physical activity should be avoided during the hours of 11 a.m. – 6 p.m. when ozone levels are particularly high.

Gusts of wind can quickly blow ozone into areas that are otherwise unexposed. However, if the nitric oxides – essential catalytic factors for the destruction of ozone – are missing in the likes of recreational areas with a low volume of traffic, ozone can remain at dangerously high levels for longer periods of time, even after sunset.

92 Sleep and health

The brain needs a sufficient amount of sleep. In this apparent resting phase, it is actually very active and regulates important body functions such as heart rate, breathing, metabolism and the immune system. Sleep is also of great importance for learning. The different sleep phases have various functions. The long-term memory necessary for specific kinds of learning, rote memorization of names, dates or learning facts, is consolidated in the deep sleep phase. By contrast, dream sleep is responsible for the procedural memory that mainly functions automatically without thinking. This covers motor processes like walking, running, swimming, jumping or riding a bicycle. Declarative and procedural capabilities are stored in different parts of the brain.

The 4 stages of sleep recorded by the electroencephalogram are the initial (falling asleep), light sleep, deep sleep (during the first half of sleep) and REM (rapid eye movement) sleep (dreaming stage). The hormone that helps regulates sleep is **melatonin**. This hormone is synthesized by the pineal gland which is located in the brain stem. The average weight of this pea-sized gland is only 0.1 g. Melatonin levels are higher in younger than in older persons. The need for sleep varies among individuals. According to data gathered by the Robert Koch Institute, the average German gets between 6 and 8 hours of sleep a night.

Chronic sleep deficits lead to markedly reduced performance during the day (Lund et al. 2010, Gildner et al. 2014).

Those affected by this disorder have a five times higher risk of becoming ill than those who get enough sleep (Cappuccio et al. 2010, 2011, Hsu et al. 2012, Laugsand et al. 2014). People suffering from chronic sleep deficit will often also suffer from high blood pressure because chronic sleep deficit adversely affects endothelial function in the large blood vessels (▶ Chapter 51) (Gangwisch et al. 2013). One particular type of sleep disorder is snoring, a condition that other fellow human beings tend to be the ones to suffer under. Nevertheless, it can also be dangerous for the snorer themselves (2 % women, 4 % men) when associated with temporary cessation of breathing (apnea). Common consequences of **sleep apnea syndrome** are high blood pressure, atrial fibrillation, myocardial infarction and stroke.

There should be a gap of two hours between the end of mental activity and going to bed. During this time, large meals should be avoided. Black and green tea, coffee, cola drinks and some painkillers contain sleep-impairing caffeine. Nicotine also has a stimulating effect and alcohol causes sleep-maintenance disorders. Physical activity is very helpful in promoting restful sleep (Brand et al. 2010). It causes tiredness and helps with falling asleep, although not immediately. Depending on the intensity level of the exercise, the body needs 2–4 hours to achieve full relaxation. Therefore, exercise should be avoided shortly before going to bed.

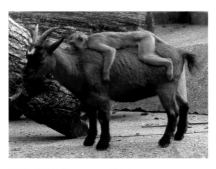

◻ Fig. 92.1 Sleep consolidates memory

93 Tobacco or health

Exercise and sports are not practiced in smoke-filled back rooms. From a health perspective, however, such a scenario of people exercising in a tobacco cloud can poignantly demonstrate how much humans depend on clean air (Strandberg et al. 2008, Yeh et al. 2010). Tobacco smoke is the most relevant toxin affecting indoor air quality in the majority of places. It is made up of the sidestream smoke that drifts from the burning end of a cigarette and the mainstream smoke exhaled by the smoker. In addition to the fine particles (▶ Chapter 90), this air pollution contains more than 7,000 chemicals of which as many as over 70 are carcinogenic. Tobacco smoke permanently changes the structure of 323 genes. The resulting damage to genetic material often triggers many smoking-related diseases. As a result of these genetic change, babies can already develop a nicotine dependence *in utero* if the mother smokes during pregnancy (Markus's et al. 2014).

Even the tiniest exposure to the substances in tobacco can lead to a heart attack. According to the results of the Cancer Prevention Study based on more than one million adults, only 3 cigarettes per day already increase the risk of a heart attack by over 60 % (Pope et al. 2009). The follow-up on nearly 4 million smokers showed that the risk of coronary heart disease is higher in women than in men (Huxley et Woodward 2011). People who have never smoked, have a mean life expectancy of 10 years longer than those dependent on tobacco (Pirie et al. 2013, Jha et al. 2013, Li et al. 2014).

Approximately one-third of all cancers in Germany are linked to smoking. This figure is consistent with data from WHO Report that one third

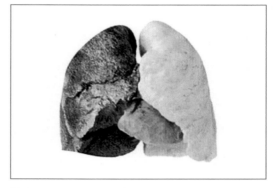

Fig. 93.1 Left and right lungs: left Smoker, right Non-smoker

of cancers could be prevented by action on smoking. Even objects contaminated by fine particulate matter from tobacco pose a continuous source of toxins, even stale tobacco smoke can damage health. Pooled meta-analyses from all previous international studies unequivocally prove that smoking is linked to the increased prevalence of:

- Acute myeloid leukemia
- Arteriosclerosis
- Chronic respiratory diseases
- Glaucoma
- Cataracts
- Coronary heart disease
- Abdominal aortic aneurysm
- Cancer of the lung, oral cavity, larynx, breast, stomach, esophagus, pancreas, kidneys, bladder, uterus and the bowel
- Gastric ulcers
- Macular degeneration

- Osteoporosis
- Rheumatoid arthritis
- Fecal incontinence in old age
- Type 2 diabetes
- Periodontitis and inflammation of the tooth root

Heavy smoking in midlife also markedly increases the risk for dementia 20 years later (Rusanen et al. 2011).

It is not only the smokers who carry all of these risks, but passive smokers are also seriously affected. Each year, around 700,000 people in the European Union and about 5.7 million worldwide die as a result. They suffer from higher rates of coronary heart disease, dementia (Chen et al. 2013) and malignant tumors. According to data from the Women's Health Initiative, women who are both active smokers and passive smokers are more likely to develop breast cancer, for example (Luo et al. 2011). According to a report by the WHO, passive smoking causes the deaths of approximately 600,000 persons worldwide each year, including 165,000 children (Öberg et al. 2011).

III Appendix

To sum up

A varied diet and plenty of exercise are critical factors for a healthy lifestyle. According to the data from large-scale international studies, a diet consisting of plenty of fruit and vegetables, restraint in eating meat and meat products, avoiding obesity, the practice of physical exercise at least 2.5 hours a week along with not smoking and moderation in the consumption of alcohol lowers the risk for serious diseases like diabetes, cancer, myocardial infarction and stroke by more than half.

The World Health Organization (WHO) currently assumes that malnutrition and lack of exercise alone are responsible for at least one-third of all diseases in western countries. According to estimates by health insurers, around 70 % of expenditures in the healthcare systems like the German one are incurred as a result of these two behavior-related factors. However, simply making people aware of these issues does not have much of an impact. It is more important, rather, for people to appreciate and assimilate the easily learned medical basics and facts to understand the consequences of potentially bad habits and behaviors. Once those affected have this knowledge and awareness, they will find it easier to successfully make lasting positive changes to their lifestyles.

Each individual not only benefits from modifications to their lifestyle and a new health consciousness by substantially raising their quality of life, but it's gentler on their pocketbook as well. Indeed, the huge progress made by biotechnology in all areas of medicine will no longer be completely funded by the tightly drawn health insurance budgets.

One particularly rewarding responsibility for adults is furthermore to be dedicated to promoting a healthy lifestyle among children and young people. True value is achieved by kindergarten and school teachers as well as the parents imparting knowledge in that they continually remind and demonstrate the importance of a healthy lifestyle in their own lives. The children then naturally and playfully assimilate the basics of a healthy lifestyle and then carry this learning with them into adulthood. If positive learning opportunities are missed, the young are already programmed with bad habits in childhood.

The ancient Greeks were long aware that

> "A simple diet, enough exercise and moderation in all things are the best ingredients for a healthy, long life."
> (Hippocrates, c. 460–370 B.C.)

> To be healthy, we need luck and knowledge. Our luck may leave us, but our knowledge remains.

Impact factors (2013)

The following table lists the specific impact factors of the medical references cited this book. The impact factor measures how often other journals mention articles from a particular academic journal in relation to the total number of original articles and reviews published. It is calculated over a two year period by adding together the number of citations, for example, made in the year 2013 by articles published in the years 2011 and 2012 and then dividing the number of citations by the total number of articles published in those two years. The higher the impact factor, the higher is the reputation of the academic journal. Out of the 151 journals evaluated, the *New England Journal of Medicine* has had the highest impact factor for many years now (◻ Table: Impact factors).

◻ **Table Impact factors (2013)**

Professional journal	Impact factor	Professional journal	Impact factor
N Engl J Med	51.658	Diabetes Care	7.735
The Lancet	39.060	Ann Oncol	7.384
Nature	38.597	Am J Clin Nutr	6.504
Nature Genetics	35.209	Mayo Clinic Proceedings	5.790
JAMA	29.978	Int J Obes	5.221
Nature Chemistry	21.757	Am J Epidemiol	4.780
BMJ	17.215	Am J Med	4.768
PLOS Med	15.253	Cancer Epidem Biom Prev	4.559
Circulation	15.202	Obesity	3.922
Eur Heart J	14.097	Arch Ophthalmol	3.826
J Am Coll Cardiol	14.086	PLOS ONE	3.730
Ann Intern Med	13.976	Brit J Sport Med	3.668
(Arch) JAMA Intern Med	11.462	Dtsch Arztebl Int	3.608
Proc Natl Acad Sci	9.809	J Epidemiol Community Health	3.392
Neurology	8.249	J Adolesc Health	2.996

Abbreviated glossary of medical terms

▪ Abbreviated glossary of medical terms

Aerobic	dependent on the presence of free oxygen
Alveolus	A small saclike structure in the lungs
Amplitude	Largeness or fullness, wideness or breadth of range or extent
Anabolic	pertaining to anabolism
Anaerobic	the absence of molecular oxygen
Angiotensin	a family of polypeptide vasopressor hormones
Antagonism	Interference with the metabolism or function of a given chemical compound
Apnea	Cessation of breathing
Arteriosclerosis	Arteriosclerosis
Arthrosis	Degenerative joint disease
Asthma	recurrent attacks of paroxysmal dyspnea, with airway inflammation and wheezing
Atherogenic	conducive to or causing atherogenesis
Bariatrics	the study of obesity, its causes, prevention, and treatment
Capillaries	minute vessels
Carcinogen	cancer-producing
Cardiomyopathy	non-inflammatory disease of the heart muscle
Cardiovascular	pertaining to the heart and blood vessels

Catecholamine	one of a group of biogenic amines having a sympathomimetic action, examples are dopamine, norepinephrine and epinephrine.
Causative	effective or responsible as a cause or agent
Chemotaxis	directional movement of an organism in response to a chemical concentration gradient
Cognitive	including all aspects of perceiving, thinking, and remembering.
Collagen	proteins occurring as a major component of connective tissue (e.g. cartilage, bone)
Concentric	having a common center
Contractility	capacity for contracting in response to a suitable stimulus
Contraction	a reduction in size or shrinkage
Contraindications	any condition which renders some particular line of treatment improper or undesirable
Convection	transmission of heat in liquids or gases
Coronary	encircling in the manner of a crown
Coronary heart disease	any of a group of acute or chronic cardiac disabilities resulting from insufficient supply of oxygenated blood to the heart
Correlation	reciprocal relationship
Cortical	pertaining to or of the nature of a cortex

Cytokines	a generic term for non-antibody proteins released by one cell population which act as intercellular mediators
Cytotoxic	damaging cells
Degenerative	causing deterioration, decline
Dementia	a general loss of cognitive abilities
Depression	a mental state of depressed mood
Deprivation	period of restriction, doing without
Diabetes mellitus	a chronic syndrome of impaired carbohydrate, protein, and fat metabolism
Diarrhea	abnormal frequency and liquidity of fecal discharges
Diverticulitis	inflammation of a diverticulum, especially inflammation related to colonic diverticula
Dysbalance	lack of balance, disequilibrium
Dysfunction	disturbance, impairment, or abnormality of the functioning of an organ
Eccentric	situated or occurring away from a center
Endogenous	growing from within the body
Endothelium	the layer of epithelial cells that lines the interior of structures such as the cavities of the heart, the lumina of blood and lymph vessels
Enzymes	protein molecules that catalyze chemical reactions of other substances
Epidemiology	the science concerned with the study of the factors determining and influencing the frequency and distribution of disease
Equivalent	Something that is essentially equal to another, or can take its place entirely
Ergometer	bicycle-like apparatus for measuring the dosed effects of exercise
Estrogens	hormones formed in the ovary
Fibrinogen	factor I in blood coagulation
Fracture	the breaking of a part, especially a bone

Genesis	the coming into being of anything; the process of originating
Genome	the entirety of the genetic information encoded by the nucleotide sequence of an organism, cell, organelle, or virus
Glaucoma	eye disease characterized by an increase in intraocular pressure
Glucagon	hormone secreted in response to hypoglycemia
Glucocorticoids	corticosteroids produced by the adrenal cortex
Glycogen	major carbohydrate reserve of animals
Gonads	Genital gland
Hemoglobin	red pigment of erythrocytes
Hepatic	pertaining to the liver
Heterocyclic	chem.: having or pertaining to a closed chain or ring formation which includes atoms of different elements
Hippocampus	Structure in lateral ventricles of the brain with a central function within the limbic system, location of the olfactory center
Hypophysis	an epithelial body located at the base of the brain
Hypothalamus	part of the diencephalon
Hypothyroidism	deficiency of thyroid activity
Immune	protected against infectious disease
Impact factor	indicator of how often other professional journals cite articles from one professional journal. The higher the impact factor (IF), the more esteemed the journal.
Insufficiency	the condition of being inadequate to perform the function
Intervention	the act or fact of interfering so as to modify
Isometric	maintaining uniform length
Kilocalorie (kcal)	unit of energy, 1 kcal = 4.15 kilojoule (kJ). In this book, kcal are converted to kJ using a rounded-down factor of 4.

Laxatives	an agent that acts to promote defecation	**Obesity**	Excessive accumulation of fat in the body
Lesion	any pathological or traumatic discontinuity of tissue or loss of function of a part	**Orthostatic**	pertaining to or caused by standing erect
Libido	sexual desire	**Osteoporosis**	reduction in bone mineral density, leading to fractures after minimal trauma
Macrophages	cells serving to ingest inhaled particulate matter found in tissues	**Ovaries**	Fallopian tubes
Medical history	Medical history of patients	**Pesticides**	poisons used to destroy pests of any sort
Melanoma	malignant tumor arising from melanocytes of the skin or other organs	**Phagocytosis**	the uptake by a cell of particulate material, such as microorganisms or cell fragments
Meta-analysis	summary of the data from primary examinations	**Phasic**	consisting of phases
Metabolism	process by which living organized substance is produced and maintained,	**Physiology**	the science of the functions of the living organism and its parts, and of the physical and chemical factors and processes involved
Metastasis	abnormal (tumor) cells distant from the site primarily involved	**Plaque**	a superficial, solid, elevated skin lesion
Mitochondrion	small spherical to rod-shaped cytoplasmic organelles, and the transformation by which energy is made available	**Plasma**	the fluid portion of the blood in which the particulate components are suspended
Monocyte	a mononuclear leukocyte	**Polycyclic**	Chem.: containing more than one molecular ring
Mortality	death rate	**Prevention**	preventive measures
Mutation	change in the genetic material	**– primary**	recommendations for a healthy lifestyle
Myeloma	a tumor composed of cells from the bone marrow	**– secondary**	measures aims to prevent disease or injury before it ever occurs (e. g., skin cancer)
Neocortex	newer portion of the cerebral cortex	**– tertiary**	the treatment of symptomatic disease in an effort to prevent its progression to disability, or premature death
Neurotransmitter	a chemical that carries messages between neurons or between neurons and muscles	**– quaternary**	prevention of unnecessary medical interventions or the prevention of overmedicalization
Newton	English physicist, 1643–1727, SI unit of force (N), 1 N is the force needed to accelerate 1 kilogram of mass at the rate of 1 m/s^2	**Pronation**	rotation of the front of the foot laterally relative to the back of the foot
Nitrosamines	any of a group of N-nitroso derivatives of secondary amines (R2N–NO)	**Prospective**	observe, look toward the futurea
Noxa(e)	an injurious agent, act, or influence	**Randomization**	assignment of experimental subjects to treatment groups according to some known probability distribution governed by chance
Nutrigenomics	a field of study combining nutrition and genomics, examining how foods affect genes		

Receptor	a sensory nerve terminal that responds to stimuli of various kinds	**Syndrome**	a set of symptoms that occur together
Rehabilitation	restoration of the ill or injured patient to optimal functional level	**Tachyarrhythmia**	any disturbance of the heart rhythm in which the heart rate is abnormally increased
Resistance	opposition, or counteracting force	**Thermogenesis**	the production of heat, especially within the animal body
Respiratory	pertaining to respiration (breathing).	**Thorax**	chest
Reversible	capable of going through a series of changes in either direction, forward or backward	**Thrombotic**	pertaining to the formation, development, or presence of a thrombus
Sensory	pertaining to or subserving sensation	**Tonic Vasomotor**	characterized by continuous muscle contraction affecting the caliber of a vessel, especially of a blood vessel
Serum	the clear portion of any body fluid		
Substitution	the act of putting one thing in the place of another	**Ventilation**	the process of exchange of air between the lungs and the environment
Supination	movements resulting in raising of the medial margin of the foot	**Ventricle**	a small, normal cavity in an organ such as the heart or brain
Symbiosis	the living together or close association of two dissimilar organisms	**Visceral Atrial fibrillation**	related to the viscera an arrhythmia in which the atria quiver continuously in a chaotic pattern
Synapse	site of functional apposition between neurons		

References

A D van der, Nooyens A, Duijnhoven F van et al. (2014) All-cause mortality risk of metabolically healthy abdominal obese individuals: the EPIC-MORGEN study. Obesity 22: 557–564

Aburto N, Ziolkovska A, Hooper L et al. (2013) Effect of lower sodium intake on health: systematic review and metaanalyses. BMJ 346: f1326

Aburto N, Hanson S, Gutierrez H et al. (2013) Effect of increased potassium intake on cardiovascular risk factors and disease: systematic review and meta-analyses. BMJ 346: f1378

Adams T, Davidson L, Litwin S et al. (2012) Health benefits of gastric bypass surgery after 6 years. JAMA 308: 1122–1131

Adams K, Leitzmann M, Ballard-Barbash R et al. (2014) Body mass and weight change in adults in relation to mortality risk. Am J Epidemiol 179: 135–144

Adamsen L, Quist M, Andersen C et al. (2009) Effect of a multimodal high intensity exercise intervention in cancer patients undergoing chemotherapy: randomized controlled trial. BMJ 339: 895–899

Adar SD, Sheppard L, Vedal S et al. (2013) Fine particulate air pollution and the progression of carotid intima-medial thickness: a prospective cohort study from the multiethnic study of atherosclerosis and air pollution. PLoS Med 10(4): e1001430

Ahlskog J, Geda Y, Graff-Radford N et al. (2011) Aerobic exercise may reduce the risk of dementia. Mayo Clinic Proceedings 86: 876–884

Aleksandrova K, Drogan D, Boeing H et al. (2014) Adiposity, mediating biomarkers and risk of colon cancer in the European prospective investigation into cancer and nutrition study. Int J Cancer 134: 612–621

Allen N, Beral V, Casabonne D et al. (2009) Moderate alcohol intake and cancer incidence in women. J Natl Cancer Inst 101: 296–305

Allen N, Siddique J, Wilkins J et al. (2014) Blood pressure trajectories in early adulthood and subclinical atherosclerosis in middle age. JAMA 311: 490–497

Ambrosini G, Bremner A, Reid A et al. (2013) No dose-dependent increase in fracture risk after long-term exposure to high doses of retinol or beta-carotene. Osteoporos Int 24: 1285–1293

Anandacoomarasamy A, Fransen M, March L (2009) Obesity and the musculoskeletal system. Curr Opin Rheumatol 21: 71–77

Andersen Z, Hvidberg M, Jensen S et al. (2011) Chronic obstructive pulmonary disease and long-term exposure to trafficrelated air pollution: a cohort study. Am J Respir Crit Care Med 183: 455–461

Andersen C, Rørth M, Ejlertsen B et al. (2013) The effects of a sixweek supervised multimodal exercise intervention during chemotherapy on cancer-related fatigue. Eur J Oncol Nurs 17: 331–339

Angeras O, Albertsson P, Karason K et al. (2013) Evidence for obesity paradox in patients with acute coronary syndromes: a report from the Swedish Coronary Angiography and Angioplasty Registry. Eur Heart J 34: 345–353

Autier P, Boniol M Pizot C et al. (2014) Vitamin D status and ill health: a systematic review. Lancet Diabetes Endocrinol 2: 76–89

Bailey D, Dresser G, Arnold J (2013) Grapefruit-medication interactions: forbidden fruit or avoidable consequences? CMAJ 185: 309–316

Bairdain S, Lien C, Stoffan A et al. (2014) A single institution's overweight pediatric population and their associated comorbid conditions. ISRN Obesity Volume 2014, Article ID 517694

Ballard-Barbash R, Friedenreich Ch, Courneya K et al. (2012) Physical activity, biomarkers and disease outcomes in cancer survivors: A systematic review. J Natl Cancer Inst 104: 815–840

Bao Y, Han J, Hu F et al. (2013) Association of nut consumption with total and cause specific mortality. N Engl J Med 369: 2001–2011

Baranski M, Srednicka-Tober D, Volakakis N et al. (2014) Higher antioxidant and lower cadmium concentrations and lower incidence of pesticide residues in organically grown crops: a systematic literature review and meta-analyses. Brit J Nutr 112: 794–811

Bateman R, Xiong C, Benzinger T et al. (2012) Clinical and biomarker changes in dominantly inherited Alzheimer's Disease. N Engl J Med 367: 795–804

Baum E, Peters K (2008) The diagnosis and treatment of primary osteoporosis according to current guidelines. Dtsch Arztebl Int 105: 573–582

Beck I, Jochner S, Gilles S et al. (2013) High environmental ozone levels lead to enhanced allergenicity of birch pollen. PLoS ONE 8(11): e80147

Beelen R, Raaschou-Nielsen O, Stafoggia M et al. (2014) Effects of long-term exposure to air pollution on natural-cause mortality: an analysis of 22 European cohorts within the multicentre ESCAPE project. Lancet 383: 785–795

Bente K (2013) Muscle as a secretory organ. Compr Physiol 3: 1337–1362

Berry J, Willis B, Gupta S et al. (2011) Lifetime risks for cardio-vascular disease mortality by cardiorespiratory fitness levels measured at ages 45, 55, and 65 years in men. J Am Coll Cardiol 57: 1604–1610

Bestwick J, Huttly W, Morris J et al. (2014) Prevention of neural tube defects: a Cross-Sectional Study of the uptake of folic acid supplementation in nearly half a million women. PLoS ONE 9(2): e89354

Bhattacharya A, Eissa N (2013) Autophagy and autoimmunity crosstalks. Front Immunol 15 (4): 88

Bibbins-Domingo K, Chertow G, Coxson P et al. (2010) Projected effect of dietary salt reductions on future cardiovascular disease. N Engl J Med 362: 590–599

Bjorge T, Engeland A, Tverdal A et al. (2008) Body mass index in adolescence in relation to cause-specific mortality: a followup of 230 000 Norwegian adolescents. Am J Epidemiol 168: 30–37

Blattmann P, Schuberth C, Pepperkok R et al. (2013) RNAibased functional profiling of loci from blood lipid genome-wide association studies identifies genes with cholesterol-regulatory function (2013). PLoS Genet 9(2): e1003338

Blencowe H, Cousens S, Modell B et al. (2010) Folic acid to reduce neonatal mortality from neural tube disorders. Int J Epidemiol 39: i110–i121

Bogers R, Bemelmans W, Hoogenveen R et al. (2007) Association of overweight with increased risk of coronary heart disease partly independent of blood pressure and cholesterol levels. Arch Intern Med 167: 1720–1728

Booth J, Leary S, Joinson C et al. (2014) Associations between objectively measured physical activity and academic attainment in adolescents from a UK cohort. Br J Sports Med 48: 265–270

Brand S, Gerber M, Beck J et al. (2010) High exercise levels are related to favorable sleep patterns and psychological functioning in adolescents: a comparison of athletes and controls. J Adolesc Health 46: 133–141

Britton K, Massaro J, Murabito J et al. (2013) Body fat distribution, incident cardiovascular disease, cancer, and all-cause mortality. J Am Coll Cardiol 62: 921–925

Brøndum-Jacobsen P, Benn M, Jensen GB et al. (2012) 25-Hydroxyvitamin D levels and risk of ischemic heart disease, myocardial infarction, and early death: Population-based study and meta-analyses of 18 and 17 studies. Arterioscler Thromb Vasc Biol 32: 2794–2802

Brouwer I, Wanders A, Katan M (2013) Trans fatty acids and cardiovascular health: research completed? Eur J Clin Nutrition 67: 541–547

Brown J, Huedo-Medina T, Pescatello L et al. (2011) Efficacy of exercise interventions in modulating cancer-related fatigue among adult cancer survivors: a meta-analysis. Cancer Epidemiol Biomarkers Prev 20: 123–133

Buckland G, Agudo A, Lujan L et al. (2010) Adherence to a mediterranean diet and risk of gastric adenocarcinoma within the European Prospective Investigation into Cancer and Nutrition (EPIC) cohort study. Am J Clin Nutr 91: 381– 390

Cahill I, Chiuve S, Mekary R et al. (2013) Prospective study of breakfast eating and incident coronary heart disease in a cohort of male US Health Professionals. Circulation 128: 337–343

Cappuccio F, D`Elia L, Strazzullo P et al. (2010) Sleep duration and all-cause mortality: a systematic review and meta-analysis of prospective studies. Sleep 33: 585–592

Cappuccio F, Cooper D, D`Elia L et al. (2011) Sleep durationpredicts cardiovascular outcomes: a systematic review and meta-analysis of prospective studies. Eur Heart J 32: 1484– 1492

Caprio S (2012) Calories from soft drinks – do they matter? N Engl J Med 367: 1462–1463

Carlsson L, Peltonen M, Ahlin S et al. (2012) Bariatric surgery and prevention of type 2 diabetes in Swedish obese subjects. N Engl J Med 367: 695–704

Carnethon M, De Chavez P, Biggs M et al. (2012) Association of weight status with mortality in adults with incident diabetes. JAMA 308: 581–590

Cassidy A, O´Reilly E, Kay C et al. (2011) Habitual intake of flavonoid subclasses and incident hypertension in adults. Am J Clin Nutr 93: 338–347

Cerhan J, Moore S, Jacobs E et al. (2014) A pooled analysis of waist circumference and mortality in 650.000 adults. Mayo Clin Proc 89: 335–345

Chen H, Goldberg M (2009) The effects of outdoor air pollution on chronic illness. Mcgill J Med 12: 58–64

Chen R, Wilson K, Chen Y et al. (2013) Association between environmental tobacco smoke exposure and dementia syndromes. Occup Environ Med 70: 63–69

Cherkas L, Hunkin J, Kato B et al. (2008) The association between physical activity in leisure time and leukocyte telomere length. Arch Intern Med 168: 154–158

Chew E (2013) Lutein + zeaxanthin and omega-3 fatty acids for age-related macular degeneration. The age-related eye disease study 2. Randomized Clinical Trial. JAMA 309: 2005–2015

Chiaranda G, Bernardi E, Codecà L et al. (2013) Treadmill walking speed and survival prediction in men with cardiovascular disease: a 10-year follow-up study. BMJ 3: e003446

Chiuve S, Sun Qi, Curhan G et al. (2013) Dietary and plasma magnesium and risk of coronary heart disease among women. J Am Heart Assoc 2: e000114

Chong E, Robman L, Simpson J et al. (2009) Fat consumption and its association with age-related macular degeneration. Arch Ophthalmol 127: 674–680

Christakis N, Fowler J (2007) The spread of obesity in a large social network over 32 years. N Engl J Med 357: 370–379

Christakis N, Fowler J (2014) Friendship and natural selection. PNAS 111: 10796–10801

Christen W, Schaumberg D, Glynn R et al. (2011) Dietary omega-3 fatty acid and fish intake and incident age-related macular degeneration in women. Arch Ophthalmol 129: 921–929

Christian M, Evans C, Hancock N et al. (2013) Family meals can help children reach their 5 a day: a cross-sectional survey of children's dietary intake from London primary schools. J Epidemiol Community Health 67: 332–338

Clarke R, Halsey J, Lewington S et al. (2010) Effects of lowering homocysteine levels with B vitamins on cardiovascular disease, cancer, and cause-specific mortality. Meta-analysis of 8 randomized trials involving 37.485 individuals. Arch Intern Med 170: 1622–1631

Cleave J van, Gortmaker S, Perrin J et al. (2010) Dynamics of obesity and chronic health conditions among children and youth. JAMA 303: 623–630

Clemson L, Singh M, Bundy A et al. (2012) Integration of balance and strength training into daily life activity to reduce rate of falls in older people (the LIFE study): randomized parallel trial. BMJ 345: e4547

Cobb L, Anderson C, Elliott P et al. (2014) Methodological issues in cohort studies that relate sodium intake to cardiovascular disease outcomes. A science advisory from the American Heart Association. Circulation 129: 1173–1186

Compston J, Cooper A, Cooper C et al. (2013) Diagnosis and management of osteoporosis in postmenopausal women and older men in the UK. National Osteoporosis Guideline Group update 2013. Maturitas 75: 392–396

Compston J, Flahive J, Hosmer D et al. (2014) Relationship of weight, height, and body mass index with fracture risk at different sites in postmenopausal women: The Global Longitudinal Study of Osteoporosis in Women (GLOW). J Bone Miner Res 29: 487–493

Cross A, Leitzmann M, Gail M et al. (2007) A prospective study of red and processed meat intake in relation to cancer risk. PloS Med 4(12): e325

Cross A, Ferrucci L, Risch et al. (2010) A large prospective study of meat consumption and colorectal cancer risk: an investigation of potential mechanisms underlying this association. Cancer Res 70: 2406–2414

Crowe K, Francis C (2013) Position of the Academy of Nutrition and Dietetics: Functional Foods. J Acad Nutr Diet 113: 1096–1103

Crowe F, Roddam A, Key T et al. (2011) Fruit and vegetable intake and mortality from ischaemic heart disease: results from the European Prospective Investigation into Cancer and Nutrition (EPIC) – Heart study. Eur Heart J 32: 1235–1243

Crowe F, Appleby P, Travis R et al. (2013) Risk of hospitalization or death from ischemic heart disease among British vegetarians and nonvegetarians: results from the EPIC-Oxford cohort study. Am J Clin Nutr 97: 597–603

Danaei G, Finucane M, Lu Y et al. (2011) National, regional, and global trends in fasting plasma glucose and diabetes prevalence since 1980: systematic analysis of health examination surveys and epidemiological studies with 370 countryyears and 2,7 million participants. Lancet 378: 31–40

David LA, Maurice CF, Carmody RN, et al. Diet rapidly and reproducibly alters the human gut microbiome. *Nature*. 2014;505(7484):559-563. doi:10.1038/nature12820.

Debette S, Baiser A, Hoffmann U et al. (2010) Visceral fat is associated with lower brain volume in healthy middle-aged adults. Ann Neurol 68: 136–144

DeFina L, Willis B, Radford N et al. (2013) The association between midlife cardiorespiratory fitness levels and laterlife dementia: a cohort study. Ann Intern Med 158: 162–168

D'Elia L, Barba G, Cappuccio et al. (2011) Potassium intake, stroke, and cardiovascular disease. J Am Coll Cardiol 57: 1210–1219

Dietz W, Scanlon K (2012) Eliminating the use of partially hydrogenated oil in food production and preparation. JAMA 308: 143–144

Djousse L, Driver J, Gaziano M (2009) Relation between modifiable lifestyle factors and lifetime risk of heart failure. JAMA 302: 394–400

Dong J, Xun P, He K et al. (2011) Magnesium intake and risk of type 2 diabetes: meta-analysis of prospective cohort studies. Diabetes Care 34: 2116–2122

Ekelund U, Luan J, Sherar L et al. (2012) Moderate to vigorous activity and sedentary time and cardiometabolic risk factors in children and adolescents. JAMA 307: 704–712

Eliassen H, Hankinson S, Rosner B et al. (2010) Physical activity and risk of breast cancer among postmenopausal women. Arch Intern Med 170: 1758–1764

ERFC (2010) Emerging Risk Factors Collaboration. Diabetes mellitus, fasting blood glucose concentration, and risk of vascular disease: a collaborative meta-analysis of 102 prospective studies. Lancet 375: 2215–2222

Farzaneh-Far R, Lin J, Epel E et al. (2010) Association of marine omega-3 fatty acid levels with telomeric aging in patients with coronary heart disease. JAMA 303: 250–257

Finucane M, Stevens G, Cowan M et al. (2011) National, regional, and global trends in body-mass index since 1980: systemic analysis of health examination surveys and epidemiological studies with 960 country-years and 9.1 million participants. Lancet 377: 557–567

Flegal K, Kit B, Orpana H et al. (2013) Association off all-cause mortality with overweight and obesity using standard body mass index categories. A systematic review and meta-analysis. JAMA 309: 71–82

Flammer A, Anderson T, Celermajer D et al. (2012) The assessment of endothelial function – from research into clinical practice. Circulation 126: 753–767

Ford E, Bergmann M, Kröger J et al. (2009) Healthy living is the best revenge. Findings from the European Prospective Investigation into Cancer and Nutrition – Potsdam study. Arch Intern Med 169: 1355–1362

Forman J, Stampfer M, Curhan G (2009) Diet and lifestyle risk factors associated with incident hypertension in women. JAMA 302: 401–411

Fung T, Rexrode K, Mantzoros C et al. (2009) Mediterranean diet and incidence of and mortality from coronary heart disease and stroke in women. Circulation 119: 1093–1100

Gangwisch J, Feskanich D, Malaspina D et al. (2013) Sleep duration and risk for hypertension in women: results from the nurses' health study. Am J Hypertens 26: 903–911

Gelber R, Petrovitch H, Masaki K et al. (2012) Lifestyle and the risk of dementia among Japanese American men. J Am Geriatr Soc 60: 118–123

Gildner T, Liebert M, Kowal P et al. (2014) Associations between sleep duration, sleep quality, and cognitive test performance among older adults from six middle income countries: results from the Study on Global Ageing and Adult Health (SAGE). J Clin Sleep Med 10: 613–621

Gonzales A, Hartge P, Cerhan J et al. (2010) Body-mass index and mortality among 1.46 million white adults. N Engl J Med 363: 2211–2219

Grammer T, Kleber M, März W et al. (2014) Low-density lipoprotein particle diameter and mortality: the Ludwigshafen Risk and Cardiovascular Health Study. Eur Heart J 16: 758– 766

Greenberg JA (2013) Obesity and early mortality in the United States. Obesity 21: 405–412

Gu Y, Nieves J, Stern Y et al. (2010) Food combination and Alzheimer disease risk. Arch Neurol 67: 699–706

Hadji P, Klein S, Gothe H et al. (2013) Epidemiologie der Osteoporose – Bone-Evaluation Study: Eine Analyse von Krankenkassen-Routinedaten. Dtsch Arztebl Int 110: 52–57

Haehling S von, Hartmann O, Anker S (2013) Does obesity make it better or worse: insights into cardiovascular illnesses. Eur Heart J 34: 330–332

Hamer M, Lavoie K, Bacon S (2014) Taking up physical activity in later life and healthy ageing: the English longitudinal study of ageing. Br J Sports Med 48: 239–243

Hammons A, Fiese B (2011) Is frequency of shared family meals related to the nutritional health of children and adolescents? Pediatrics 127: 1565–1574

Hanada R, Leibbrandt A, Hanada T et al. (2009) Central control of fever and female body temperature by RANKL/RANK. Nature 462: 505–509

Hardoon S, Morris R, Whincup P et al. (2012) Rising adiposity curbing decline in the incidence of myocardial infarction: 20-year follow-up of British men and women in the Whitehall II cohort. Eur Heart J 33: 478–485

He G, Luo W, Li P et al. (2010) Gamma-secretase activating protein is a therapeutic target for Alzheimer's disease. Nature 467: 95–98

He K, Du S, Xun P et al. (2011) Consumption of monosodium glutamate in relation to incidence of overweight in Chinese adults: China Health and Nutrition Survey (CHNS). Am J Clin Nutr 93: 1328–1336

Heid I, Jackson A, Randall C et al. (2010) Meta-analysis identifies 13 new loci associated with waist-hip ratio and reveals sexual dimorphism in the genetic basis of fat distribution. Nature Genetics 42: 949–960

Hildebrand J, Gapstur S, Campbell P et al. (2013) Recreational physical activity and leisure-time sitting in relation to postmenopausal breast cancer risk. Cancer Epidemiol Biomarkers Prev 22(10): 1906–1912

Hooper L, Abdelhamid A, Moore H et al. (2012) Effect of reducing total fat intake on body weight: systematic review and meta-analysis of randomised controlled trials and cohort studies. BMJ 345: e7666

Hruby A, Meigs J, O'Donnell C et al. (2014) Higher magnesium intake reduces risk of impaired glucose and insulin metabolism and progression from prediabetes to diabetes in middle-aged Americans. Diabetes Care 37: 2419–2427

Hsia J, Larson J, Ockene J et al. (2009) Resting heart rate as a low tech predictor of coronary events in women: prospective cohort study. BMJ 338: b219

Hsu C, Huang C, Huang P et al. (2012) Insomnia and risk of cardiovascular disease. Circulation 126: A15883

Huxley R, Woodward M (2011) Cigarette smoking as a risk factor for coronary heart disease in women compared with men: a systematic review and meta-analysis of prospective cohort studies. Lancet 378: 1297–1305

Jackson C, Herber-Gast G, Brown W (2014) Joint effects of physical activity and bmi on risk of hypertension in women: a longitudinal study. J Obes 2014: 271532

Jafri H, Alsheikh-Ali A, Karas R (2010) Baseline and on-treatment high-density lipoprotein cholesterol and the risk of cancer in randomized controlled trials of lipid-altering therapy. J Am Coll Cardiol 55: 2846–2854

Jenab M, Bueno-de-Mesquita B, Ferrari P et al. (2010) Association between pre-diagnostic circulating vitamin D concentration and risk of colorectal cancer in European populations: a nested case-control study. BMJ 340: b5500

Jerrett M, Burnett R, Pope A et al. (2009) Long-term ozone exposure and mortality. N Engl J Med 360: 1085–1095

Jha P, Ramasundarahettige C, Landsman V et al. (2013) 21st-century hazards of smoking and benefits of cessation in the United States. N Engl J Med 368: 341–350

Kamstrup P, Tybjærg-Hansen A, Nordestgaard B (2013) Extreme Lipoprotein(a) levels and improved cardiovascular risk prediction. J Am Coll Cardiol 61: 1146–1156

Kantomaa M, Stamatakis E, Kaakinen M et al. (2013) Physical activity and obesity mediate the association between childhood motor function and adolescents' academic achievement. Proc Natl Acad Sci 110: 1917–1922

Kastorini CM, Milionis H, Esposito K et al. (2011) The effect of mediterranean diet on metabolic syndrome and its components. J Am Coll Cardiol 57: 1299–1313

Keszei A, Schouten L, Goldbohm R et al. (2012) Red and processed meat consumption and the risk of esophageal and gastric cancer subtypes in The Netherlands Cohort Study. Ann Oncol 23: 2319–2326

Khan N, Afag F, Mukhtar H (2010) Lifestyle and risk factor for cancer: Evidence from human studies. Cancer Lett 293: 133–143

Khera A, Cuchel M, Liera-Moya M et al. (2011) Cholesterol efflux capacity, high-density lipoprotein function, and atherosclerosis. N Engl J Med 364: 127–135

Kim D, Xun P, Liu K et al. (2010) Magnesium intake in relation to systemic inflammation, insulin resistence, and the incidence of diabetes. Diabetes Care 33: 2604–2610

Kim MS, Pinto SM, Getnet D et al. (2014) A draft map of the human proteome. Nature 509: 575–581

Kodoma S, Saito K, Tanaka S et al. (2011) Alcohol consumption and risk of atrial fibrillation. J Am Coll Cardiol 57: 427– 436

Koerte I, Ertl-Wagner B, Reiser M et al. (2012) White matter integrity in the brains of professional soccer players without a symptomatic concussion. JAMA 308: 1859–1861

Krakauer N, Krakauer J (2014) Dynamic association of mortality hazard with body shape. PLoS ONE 9(2): e88793. doi:10.1371

Kvaavik E, Batty D, Ursin G et al. (2010) Influence of individual and combined health behaviours on total and cause-specific mortality in men and women. Arch Intern Med 170: 711–718

Larsen T, Dalskov S, van Baak M et al. (2010) Diets with high or low protein content and glycemic index for weight-loss maintenance. N Engl J Med 363: 2102–2113

Larson E, Clair J, Sumner W et al. (2013) Depressed pacemaker activity of sinoatrial node myocytes contributes to the age-dependent decline in maximum heart rate. PNAS 110: 18011–18016

Laugsand L, Strand L, Platou C et al. (2014) Insomnia and the risk of incident heart failure: a population study. Eur Heart J 35 (21): 1382–1393

Lee Y, Derakhshan M (2013) Environmental and lifestyle risk factors of gastric cancer. Arch Iran Med 16: 358–365

Lee P, Swarbrick M, Ho K (2013) Brown adipose tissue in adult humans: a metabolic renaissance. Endocr Rev 34: 413–438

Leenders M, Sluijs I, Ros MM et al. (2013) Fruit and vegetable consumption and mortality: European prospective investigation into cancer and nutrition. Am J Epidemiol 178: 590–602

Leitzmann M, Moore S, Peters T et al. (2008) Prospective study of physical activity and risk of postmenopausal breast cancer. Breast Cancer Research 10: R92

Leyk D (2009) Bedeutung regelmäßiger körperlicher Aktivitäten in Prävention und Therapie. Dtsch Arztebl Int 106: 713–714

Li K, Hüsing A, Kaaks R (2014) Lifestyle risk factors and residual life expectancy at age 40: a German cohort study. BMC Medicine 12: 59

Li S, Shin H, Ding E et al.(2009) Adiponectin levels and risk of type 2 diabetes: a systematic review and meta-analysis. JAMA 302: 179–188

Liebermann D, Venkadesan M, Werbel W et al. (2010) Foot strike patterns and collision forces in habitually barefoot versus shod runners. Nature 463: 531–536

Llewellyn D, Lang I, Langa K et al. (2010) Vitamin D and risk of cognitive decline in elderly persons. Arch Intern Med 170: 1135–1141

Lloyd-Jones D, Goff D, Stone N (2014) Statins, risk assessment, and the new American prevention guidelines. Lancet 383: 600–602

Lu Y, Hajifathalian K, Ezzati M et al. (2014) Metabolic mediators of the effects of body-mass index, overweight, and obesity on coronary heart disease and stroke: a pooled analysis of 97 prospective cohorts with 1·8 million participants. Lancet 383: 970–983

Lund H, Reider B, Whiting A et al. (2010) Sleep patterns and predictors of disturbed sleep in a large population of college students. J Adolesc Health 46: 124–132

Luo J, Margolis K, Wactawski-Wende J et al. (2011) Association of active and passive smoking with risk of breast cancer among postmenopausal women: a prospective cohort study. BMJ 342: d1016

Mancia G, Fagard R, Narkiewicz K et al. (2013) ESH/ESC Guidelines for the management of arterial hypertension. J Hypertension 31: 1281–1357

Marijon E, Bougouin W, Périer MC et al. (2013) Incidence of sports-related sudden death in France by specific sports and sex. JAMA 310: 642–643

Markunas C, Xu Z, Harlid S et al. (2014) Identification of DNA methylation changes in newborns related to maternal smoking during pregnancy. Environ Health Perspect. 122: 1147–1153

Maruti S, Willett W, Feskanich D et al. (2008) A prospective study of age-specific physical activity and premenopausal breast cancer. J Nat Cancer Inst 100: 728–737

McAllister T, Ford J, Flashman L et al. (2014) Effect of head impacts on diffusivity measures in a cohort of collegiate contact sport athletes. Neurology 82: 63–69

Mensink G, Schienkiewitz A, Haftenberger M et al. (2013) Übergewicht und Adipositas in Deutschland. Ergebnisse der Studie zur Gesundheit Erwachsener in Deutschland (DEGS1). Bundesgesundheitsblatt 56: 786–794

Micha R, Mozaffarian D (2009) Trans fatty acids: effects on metabolic syndrome, heart disease and diabetes. Nature Rev Endocrinol 5: 335–344

Micha R, Wallace S, Mozaffarian D (2010) Red and processed meat consumption and risk of coronary heart disease, stroke, and diabetes mellitus. A systematic review and meta-analysis. Circulation 121: 2271–2283

Michaelsson K, Melhus H, Warensjö E et al. (2013) Long term calcium intake and rates of all cause and cardiovascular mortality: community based prospective longitudinal cohort study. BMJ 346: f228

Middleton L, Barnes D, Lui L et al. (2010) Physical activity over the life course and its association with cognitive performance and impairment in old age. J Am Geriatr Soc 58: 1322–1326

Mitrou P, Kipnis V, Thiebaut A et al. (2007) Mediterranean dietary pattern and prediction of all-cause mortality in a US population. Arch Intern Med 167: 2461–2468

Moore S, Patel A, Matthews C et al. (2012) Leisure time physical activity of moderate to vigorous intensity and mortality: a large pooled cohort analysis. PloS Med 9: e1001335

Mozaffarian D, Fahimi S, Singh G et al. (2014) Global sodium consumption and death from cardiovascular causes. N Engl J Med 371: 624–634

Mursu J, Robien K, Harnack L et al. (2011) Dietary supplements and mortality rate in older women. Arch Intern Med 171: 1625–1633

Naci H, Ioannidis J (2013) Comparative effectiveness of exercise and drug interventions on mortality outcomes: metaepidemiological study. BMJ 347: f5577

Nauman J, Nilsen T, Wisloff U et al. (2010) Combined effect of resting heart rate and physical activity on ischaemic heart disease: mortality follow-up in a population study (the HUNT study, Norway). J Epidemiol Community Health 64: 175–181

Neal D, Wood W, Drolet A (2013) How do people adhere to goals when willpower is low? The profits (and pitfalls) of strong habits. J Personality Soc Psychol 104: 959–975

Neuhouser M, Wassertheil-Smoller S, Thomson C et al. (2009) Multivitamin use and risk of cancer and cardiovascular disease in the women's health initiative cohorts. Arch Intern Med 169: 294–304

Neumann B, Walter T, Heriche J-K et al. (2010) Phenotypic profiling of the human genome by time-lapse microscopy reveals cell division genes. Nature 464: 721–727

Ng M, Fleming T, Robinson M et al. (2014) Global, regional, and national prevalence of overweight and obesity in children and adults during 1980-2013: a systematic analysis for the Global Burden of Disease Study 2013. Lancet 384: 766–781

Nguyen A, Herzog H, Sainsbury A (2011) Neuropeptide Y and peptide YY: important regulators of energy metabolism. Curr Opin Endocrinol Diabetes Obesity 18: 56–60

Nordström P, Nordström A, Eriksson M et al. (2013) Risk factors in late adolescence for young-onset dementia in men: a nationwide cohort study. JAMA Intern Med 173: 1612–1618

Öberg M, Jaakkola M, Woodward A et al. (2011) Worldwide burden of disease from exposure to second-hand smoke: a retrospective analysis of data from 192 coutries. Lancet 377: 139–146

O'Brien P, MacDonald L, Anderson M et al. (2013) Long-term outcomes after bariatric: fifteen -year followup of adjustable gastric banding and a systematic review of the bariatric surgical literature. Ann Surg 257: 87–94

Ogden C, Carroll M, Kit B et al. (2012) Prevalence of obesity and trends in body mass index among US children and adolescents, 1999-2010. JAMA 307: 483–490

Oh J, Lee H (2012) Modulation of pathogen recognition by autophagy. Front Immunol 12 (3): 44

Oyebode O, Gordon-Dseagu V, Walker A et al. (2014) Fruit and vegetable consumption and all-cause, cancer and CVD mortality: analysis of Health Survey for England data. J Epidemiol Community Health 68: 856–862

Page K, Chan O, Arora J et al. (2013) Effects of fructose vs glucose on regional cerebral blood flow in brain regions involved with appetite and reward pathways. JAMA 309: 63–70

Pan A, Sun Qi, Bernstein A et al. (2011) Red meat consumption and risk of type 2 diabetes: 3 cohorts of US adults and an updated meta-analysis. Am J Clin Nutr 94: 1–9

Pan A, Sun Q, Bernstein A et al. (2013) Changes in red meat consumption and subsequent risk of type 2 diabetes mellitus: Three cohorts of US men and women. JAMA Intern Med 173: 1328–1335

Park Y, Subar A, Hollenbeck A et al. (2011) Dietary fiber intake and mortality in the NIH-AARP Diet and Health Study. Arch Intern Med 171: 1061–1068

Parker J, Hashmi O, Dutton D et al. (2010) Levels of vitamin D and cardiometabolic disorders: systematic review and meta-analysis. Maturitas 65: 225–236

Paul C, Au R, Fredman L et al. (2008) Association of alcohol consumption with brain volume in the Framingham Study. Arch Neurol 65: 1363–1367

Pedersen B, Febbraio M (2012) Muscles, exercise and obesity: skeletal muscle as a secretory organ. Nat Rev Endocrinol 8: 457–465

Peterlik M, Grant W, Cross H (2009) Calcium, vitamin D and cancer. Anticancer Res 29: 3687–3698

Peters T, Schatzkin A, Gierach G et al. (2009) Physical activity and postmenopausal breast cancer risk in the NIH-AARP Diet and Health Study. Cancer Epidemiol Biomarkers Prev 18: 289–296

Pirie K, Peto R, Reeves G et al. (2013) The 21st century hazards of smoking and benefits of stopping: a prospective study of one million women in the UK. Lancet 381: 133–141

Pirmohamed M (2013) Drug-grapefruit juice interactions. BMJ 346: f1

Ploeg H van der, Chey T, Korda R et al. (2012) Sitting time and all-cause mortality risk in 222.497 Australian adults. Arch Intern Med 172: 494–500

Pope C, Burnett R, Krewski D et al. (2009) Cardiovascular mortality and exposure to airborne fine particulate matter and cigarette smoke. Circulation 120: 941–948

Prüss-Ustün A, Vickers C, Haefliger P et al. (2011) Knowns and unknowns on burden of disease due to chemicals: a systematic review. Environ Health 10: 9

Pschyrembel (2014) Klinisches Wörterbuch. 266., neu bearb. Aufl. 2015, De Gruyter, Berlin

Raaschou-Nielsen O, Andersen Z, Beelen R et al. (2013) Air pollution and lung cancer incidence in 17 European cohorts: prospective analyses from the European Study of Cohorts for Air Pollution Effects (ESCAPE). Lancet Oncol 14: 813– 822

Rasmussen-Torvik L, Shay Ch, Abramson J et al. (2013) Ideal cardiovascular health is inversely associated with incident cancer – the atherosclerosis risk in communities study. Circulation 127: 1270–1275

Renehan A, Tyson M, Egger M et al. (2008) Body-mass index and incidence of cancer: a systematic review and meta-analysis of prospective observational studies. Lancet 371: 569–578

Ristow M, Zarse K, Oberbach A et al. (2009) Antioxidants prevent health-promoting effects of physical exercise in humans. Proc Natl Acad Sci 106: 8665–8670

Ritz E, Hahn K, Ketteler M et al. (2012) Gesundheitsrisiko durch Phosphatzusätze in Nahrungsmitteln. Dtsch Arztebl Int 109: 49–55

Rock C, Doyle C, Demark-Wahnefried W et al. (2012) Nutrition and physical activity guidelines for cancer survivors. CA Cancer J Clin 62: 243–274

Rohrmann S, Overvad K, Bueno-de-Mesquita H et al. (2013) Meat consumption and mortality – results from the European Prospective Investigation into Cancer and Nutrition. BMC Med 11: 63

Romero-Corral A, Sert-Kuniyoshi F, Sierra-Johnson J et al. (2010) Modest visceral fat gain causes endothelial dysfunction in healthy humans. J Am Coll Cardiol 56: 662–666

Roncaglioni M, Negri M, Tombesi M et al. (2013) n–3 fatty acids in patients with multiple cardiovascular risk factors – The Risk and Prevention Study Collaborative Group. N Engl J Med 368: 1800–1808

Rubinsztein D, Shpilka T, Elazar Z (2012) Mechanisms of autophagosome biogenesis. Curr Biol 22: R29–R34

Ruiz-Canela M, Estruch R, Corella D et al. (2014) Association of mediterranean diet with peripheral artery disease: the PREDIMED randomized trial. JAMA 311: 415–417

Rusanen M, Kivipelto M, Quesenberry C et al. (2011) Heavy smoking in midlife and long-term risk of Alzheimer disease and vascular dementia. Arch Intern Med 171: 333– 339

Ruyter J de, Olthof M, Seidell J et al. (2012) Trial of sugar-free or sugar-sweetened beverages and body weight in children. N Engl J Med 367: 1397–1406

Sabate J, Oda K, Ros E (2011) Nut consumption and blood lipid levels. A pooled analysis of 25 intervention trials. Arch Intern Med 170: 821–827

Sales N, Pelegrini P, Goersch M (2014) Nutrigenomics: Definitions and advances of this new science. J Nutr Metab. ID 202759

Sanchez-Villegas A, Verbene L, De Irala J et al. (2011) Dietary fat intake and the risk of depression: the SUN project. PloS ONE 6(1): e16268

Satterthwaite T, Shinohara R, Wolf D et al. (2014) Impact of puberty on the evolution of cerebral perfusion during adolescence. PNAS 111: 8643–8648

Schmid D, Leitzmann M (2014) Television viewing and time spent sedentary in relation to cancer risk: a meta-analysis. J Natl Cancer Inst 106 (7): dju098

Schnohr P, Marott J, Lange P et al. (2013) Longevity in male and female joggers: the Copenhagen City Heart Study. Am J Epidemiol 177: 683–689

Schöttker B, Haug U, Schomburg L et al. (2013) Strong associations of 25-hydroxyvitamin D concentrations with all-cause, cardiovascular, cancer, and respiratory disease mortality in a large cohort study. Am J Clin Nutr 97: 782–793

Schulze M, Schulz M, Heidemann C et al. (2007) Fiber and magnesium intake and incidence + 29 of typ 2 diabetes. Arch Intern Med 167: 956–965

Schürks M, Glynn R, Rist P et al. (2010) Effects of vitamin E on stroke subtypes: meta-analysis of randomised controlled trials. BMJ 341:c5702

Schutter A de, Lavie C, Kachur S et al. (2014) Body composition and mortality in a large cohort with preserved ejection fraction: untangling the obesity paradox. Mayo Clinic Proc 89: 1072–1079

Schütze M, Boeing H, Pischon T et al. (2011) Alcohol attributable burden of incidence of cancer in eight European countries based on results from prospective cohort study. BMJ 342:d1584

Shah A, Langrish J, Nair H et al. (2013) Global association of air pollution and heart failure: a systematic review and metaanalysis. Lancet 382: 1039–1048

Sharma A, Vallakati A, Einstein A et al. (2014) Relationship of body mass index with total mortality, cardiovascular mortality, and myocardial infarction after coronary revascularization: evidence from a meta-analysis. Mayo Clin Proc 89 (8): 1080–1100

Shiraiwa M, Sosedova Y, Rouvie`re A et al. (2011) The role of long-lived reactive oxygen intermediates in the reaction of ozone with aerosol particles. Nature Chemistry 3: 291–295

Sinha R, Cross A, Graubard B et al. (2009) Meat intake and mortality: a prospective study of over half a million people. Arch Intern Med 169: 562–571

Sjöström L, Narbro K, Sjöström D et al. (2007) Effects of bariatric surgery on mortality in Swedish obese subjects. N Engl J Med 357: 741–752

Sjöström et al. (2012) Bariatric surgery reduces long-term cardiovascular risk in diabetes patients. JAMA 307: 56–65

Sjöström L, Peltonen M, Jacobson P et al. (2014) Association of bariatric surgery with long-term remission of type 2 diabetes and with microvascular and macrovascular complications. JAMA 311: 2297–2304

Sluijs I, van der Schouw Y, Spijkerman A et al. (2010) Carbohydrate quantity and quality and risk of type 2 diabetes in the European Prospective Investigation into Cancer and NutritionNetherlands (EPIC-NL) study. Am J Clin Nutr 92: 905–911

Smith C, Nielson K, Woodard J et al. (2014) Physical activity reduces hippocampal atrophy in elders at genetic risk for Alzheimer's disease. Front Aging Neurosci 6: 61

Smith S, Sumar B, Dixon K (2014) Musculoskeletal pain in overweight and obese children. Int J Obesity 38: 11–15

Sofi F, Cesari F, Abbate R et al. (2008) Adherence to mediterranean diet and health status: meta-analysis. BMJ 337: a1344

Sorensen M, Chi T, Shara N et al. (2014) Activity, energy intake, obesity, and the risk of incident kidney stones in postmenopausal women: a report from the Women's Health Initiative. J Am Soc Nephrol 25: 362–369

Speliotes E, Willer C, Berndt S et al. (2010) Association analyses of 249.796 individuals reveal 18 new loci associated with body mass index. Nature Genetics 42: 937–948

Stessman J, Hammerman-Rotzenberg R, Cohen A et al. (2009) Physical activity, function, and longevity among the very old. Arch Intern Med 169: 1476–1483

Stone N, Robinson J, Lichtenstein A et al. (2014) ACC/AHA Guideline on the treatment of blood cholesterol to reduce atherosclerotic cardiovascular risk in adults: a report of the American College of Cardiology/American Heart Association task force on practice guidelines. Circulation 129: S 1 – S 49

Strandberg A, Strandberg E, Pitkälä K et al. (2008) The effect of smoking in midlife on health-related quality of life in old age. A 26-year prospective study. Arch Intern Med 168: 1968–1974

Strate L, Liu Y, Aldoori W et al. (2009) Obesity increases the risk of diverticulitis and diverticular bleeding. Gastro-enterology 136: 115–122

Strazzullo P, D`Elia L, Kandala N et al. (2009) Salt intake, stroke, and cardiovascular disease: meta-analysis of prospective studies. BMJ 339:b4567

Studenski S, Perera S, Patei K et al. (2011)Gait speed and survival in older adults. JAMA 305: 50–58

Sun Qi, Townsend M, Okereke O et al. (2009) Adiposity and weight change in mid-life in relation to healthy survival after age 70 in women: prospective cohort study. BMJ 339:b3796

Sun Qi, Spiegelman D, van Dam R et al. (2010) White rice, brown rice, and risk of type 2 diabetes in US men and women. Arch Intern Med 170: 961–969

Sun Q, Shi L, Prescott J et al. (2012) Healthy lifestyle and leukocyte telomere length in U.S. women. Plos One 7(5):e38374

Sundström J, Neovius M, Tynelius P et al. (2011) Association of blood pressure in late adolescence with subsequent mortality: cohort study of Swedish male conscripts. BMJ 342:d643

Swardfager W, Herrmann N, Cornish S et al. (2012) Exercise intervention and inflammatory markers in coronary artery disease: a meta-analysis. Am Heart J 163: 666–676

Te Morenga L, Mallard S, Mann J (2013) Dietary sugars and body weight: systematic review and meta-analyses of randomised controlled trials and cohort studies. BMJ 346:e7492

Tomkinson G (2013) American Heart Association meeting report in Dallas 2013: Abstract 13498

Tonne C, Wilkinson P (2013) Long-term exposure to air pollu-tion is associated with survival following acute coronary syndrome. Eur Heart J 34: 1306–1311

Tsivgoulis G, Judd S, Letter A et al. (2013) Adherence to a Mediterranean diet and risk of incident cognitive impairment. Neurology 80: 1684–1692

Vaag A (2009) Neuroendocrine, metabolic and pharmacologi-cal control of feeding behavior – closing in on antiobesity treatment. J Physiol 587: 17–18

Vestergaard P, Rejnmark L, Mosekilde L (2010) High-dose treatment with vitamin A analogues and risk of fractures. Arch Dermatol 146: 478–482

Wada K, Nagata C, Tamakoshi A et al. (2014) Body mass index and breast cancer risk in Japan: a pooled analysis of eight population-based cohort studies. Ann Oncol 25: 519–524

Wang Y, Sympson J, Wluka A et al. (2009) Relationship be-tween body adiposity measures and risk of primary knee and hip replacement for osteoarthritis: a prospective cohort study. Arthritis Res Ther 11:R31

Wang X, Ouyang Y, Liu J et al. (2014) Fruit and vegetable consumption and mortality from all causes, cardiovas-cular disease, and cancer: systematic review and dose-response meta-analysis of prospective cohort studies. BMJ 349: g4490

Wen CP, Wai J, Tsai M et al. (2011) Minimum amount of physical activity for reduced mortality and extended life expec-tancy: a prospective cohort study. Lancet 378: 1244–1253

Westerterp K (2013) Physical activity and physical activity induced energy expenditure in humans: measurement, determinants, and effects. Front Physiol 4: 90

West-Wright C, Henderson K, Sullivan-Halley J et al. (2009) Long-term and recent recreational physical activity and survival after breast cancer: the California Teachers Study. Cancer Epidemiol Biomarkers Prev 18: 2851–2859

Whitmer RA, Gustafson DR, Barrett-Connor E et al. (2008) Central obesity and increased risk of dementia more than three decades later. Neurology 71: 1057–1064

Whitlock G, Lewington S, Sherliker P et al. (2009) Body-mass index and cause-specific mortality in 900.000 adults: collaborative analyses of 57 prospective studies. Lancet 373: 1083–1096

WHO (2009) World Health Organization/FAO (Food and Agri-culture Organization). WHO/FAO release independent expert report on diet and chronic disease, 2009. http://www.who. int/mediacentre/news/releases/2003/pr20/en. Accessed on 10 August 2014

WHO (2014) World Health Organization. WHO – Physical activity and adults. Recommended levels of physical activity for adults aged 18– 64 years. http://www.who.int/dietphysicalactivity/factsheet/adults/en. Accessed on 10 August 2014

WHO (2016) World Health Organization. WHO – Health Topics, Aging. http://www.who.int/topics/ageing/en/. Accessed on 21 January 2016

WHO (2016) World Health Organization. WHO – Media centre, Dementia. http://www.who.int/mediacentre/factsheets/fs362/en/. Accessed on 21 January 2016

WHO (2016) World Health Organization. WHO – Media centre, Global cancer rates could increase by 50% to 15 million by 2020. http://www.who.int/mediacentre/news/releases/2003/pr27/en/. Accessed on 21 January

Wijngaarden J van, Doets E, Szczecińska A et al. (2013) Vitamin B12, Folate, Homocysteine, and bone health in adults and elderly people: a systematic review with meta-analyses. J Nutr Metab 2013: 486186

Wilhelm M, Schlegl J, Hahne H et al. (2014) Mass-spectro-metrybased draft of the human proteome. Nature 509: 582–587

Willeit P, Willeit J, Mayr A et al. (2010) Telomere length and risk of incident cancer and cancer mortality. JAMA 304: 69–75

Wilmot EG, Edwardson CL, Achana FA et al. (2012) Sedentary time in adults and the association with diabetes, cardio-vascular disease and death: Systematic review and meta-analysis. Diabetologia 55: 2895–2905

Wiskemann J, Steindorf K (2013) Sportund Bewegungs-therapie in der Onkologie – Positive Einflüsse auf Tumorprogression und Überlebensraten. Klinikarzt 42: 402–405

Wolin K, Yan Y, Colditz G (2011) Physical activity and risk of colon adenoma: a meta-analysis. Br J Cancer 104: 882–885

World Cancer Research Fund (2009) American Institute for Cancer Research. Food, Nutrition, Physical Activity, and the Prevention of Cancer. A global perspective. ACIR, Washington DC

Xiao Q, Murphy R, Houston D et al. (2013) Dietary and supple-mental calcium intake and cardiovascular disease mortal-ity: the National Institutes of Health-AARP diet and health study. JAMA Intern Med 173: 639–646

Xu W, Atti A, Gatz M et al. (2011) Midlife overweight and obesity increase late-life dementia risk. A population-based twin study. Neurology 76: 1568–1574

Yaghootkar H, Lamina C, Scott R et al. (2013) Mendelian randomization studies do not support a causal role for reduced circulating adiponectin levels in insulin resis-tance and type 2 diabetes. Diabetes 62: 3589–3598

Yamada Y, Noriyasu R, Yokoyama K et al. (2013) Association between lifestyle and physical activity level in the elderly: a study using doubly labeled water and simplified physi-cal activity record. Eur J Appl Physiol 113: 2461–2471

Yao B, Fang H, Xu W et al. (2014) Dietary fiber intake and risk of type 2 diabetes: a dose–response analysis of prospec-tive studies. Eur J Epidemiol 29: 79–88

Yeh H, Duncan B, Schmidt M et al. (2010) Smoking, smoking cessation, and risk for typ 2 diabetes mellitus – a cohort study. Ann Intern Med 152: 10–17

Yeung E, Zhang C, Willett W et al. (2010) Childhood size and life course weight characteristics in association with the risk of incident type 2 diabetes. Diabetes Care 33: 1364–1369

Yokoyama Y, Nishimura K, Barnard N et al. (2014) Vegetarian diets and blood pressure. A meta-analysis. JAMA Intern Med 174: 577–587

Yuan C, Bao Y, Wu C et al. (2013) Prediagnostic body mass index and pancreatic cancer survival. J Clin Oncol 31: 4229–4234

Zamora-Ros R, Forouhi N, Sharp S et al. (2014) Dietary intakes of individual flavanols and flavonols are inversely asso-ciated with incident type 2 diabetes in European popula-tions. J Nutr 144: 335–343

Zaridze D, Lewington S, Boroda A et al. (2014) Alcohol and mortality in Russia: prospective observational study of 151 000 adults. Lancet 383: 1465–1473

Zhang C, Rexrode K, Dam R van et al. (2008) Abdominal obesity and risk of all-cause, cardiovascular, and cancer mortality. Circulation 117: 1658–1667

Zheng W, Lee S (2009) Well-done meat intake, heterocyclic amine exposure, and cancer risk. Nutr Cancer 61: 437–446

Printed in the United States
By Bookmasters